Pocket Companion for

Critical
Care
Nursing

Pocket Companion for

Critical Care Nursing

Sheila Melander, DSN, RN, FCCM
Associate Professor of Nursing
University of Southern Indiana
Evansville, Indiana

Linda Bucher, DNSc, RN
Associate Professor of Nursing
University of Delaware
Newark, Delaware

W.B. SAUNDERS COMPANY
A Division of Harcourt Brace & Company
Philadelphia London Toronto Montreal Sydney Tokyo

W.B. SAUNDERS COMPANY
A Division of Harcourt Brace & Company

The Curtis Center
Independence Square West
Philadelphia, Pennsylvania 19106

Library of Congress Cataloging-in-Publication Data

Melander, Sheila Drake.
Pocket companion for critical care nursing/Sheila Melander,
Linda Bucher.—1st ed.

p.   cm.

ISBN 0–7216–6919–0

1. Intensive care nursing—Handbooks, manuals, etc.
   I. Bucher, Linda.   II. Title.   [DNLM: 1. Critical Care
   nurses' instruction handbooks.   2. Critical Illness—
   nursing handbooks.   WY 49 M517p 1999]

RT120.I5M468   1999   610.73′61—dc21

DNLM/DLC   98–43361

Pocket Companion for
Critical Care Nursing   ISBN   0–7216–6919–0

Copyright © 1999 by W.B. Saunders Company

Printed in the United States of America

Last digit is the print
number: 9   8   7   6   5   4   3   2   1

Preface

The purpose of the *Pocket Companion for Critical Care Nursing* is to provide the practicing critical care nurse and the critical care nursing student with a portable, quick-reference handbook that can be used at the patient's bedside. It is designed to include critical care concepts related to each body system, including anatomy and physiology and physical assessment. Technologic devices, laboratory and diagnostic tests with normal values, and specific disease states are included. Figures, tables, and charts are adapted from the more extensive *Critical Care Nursing* text (edited by Linda Bucher and Sheila Melander) for fingertip accessibility and ease of reference.

The critical care environment includes diverse patients who evidence complex, highly specialized needs and extensive co-morbidity and who require sophisticated technology. To provide a high quality of patient care, nurses must maintain a high level of knowledge and competency and consult appropriate resources as needed. We hope that you find this handbook informative, readable, current, and useful in your daily practice, and that it assists you in meeting the challenges of critical care nursing.

Table of Contents

Multisystem Disorders   461

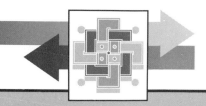

Cardiovascular
System

Cardiovascular Anatomy and Physiology

Normal Heart Cross Section

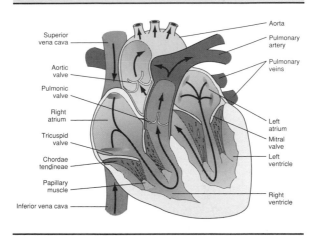

The Cardiac Cycle

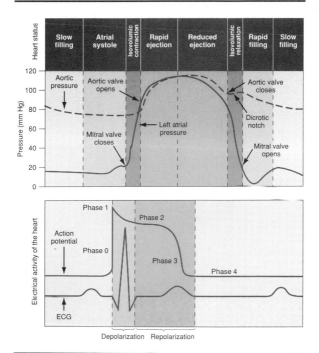

Hemodynamic Parameters

PARAMETER	NORMAL	FORMULA	CAUSES OF HIGH VALUES	CAUSES OF LOW VALUES
Cardiac index (CI)	2.5–4.0 L/min/m²	CO/BSA	Sepsis (due to peripheral vasodilation)	Abnormal heart rate ↓Contractility ↓Preload ↑Afterload
Cardiac output (CO)	4–8 L/min	HR × SV	Sepsis (due to peripheral vasodilation)	Abnormal heart rate ↓Contractility ↓Preload ↑Afterload
Central venous pressure/right atrial pressure (CVP/RAP)	2–6 cm H_2O 2–8 mm Hg		Fluid overload, venous constriction, pulmonary hypertension	Dehydration, diuretics, hemorrhage venodilation, third spacing, dysrhythmias

Parameter	Normal value	Formula		
Left ventricular stroke work index (LVSWI)	40–70 g/m²/beat	$$\frac{(MAP - PAD)}{CI} \, SV \times .0136$$	Response to catecholamines (beta stimulants, milrinone), normal electrolyte levels, aerobic metabolism, <40% loss of functional myocardium, increased preload	Myocardial infarction, drugs (beta blockers, calcium channel blockers), hyponatremia, hyperkalemia, anaerobic metabolism, >40% loss of functional myocardium, decreased preload, myocardial depressant factor
Mean arterial pressure (MAP)	70–105 mm Hg	$$\frac{SBP + (2 \times DBP)}{3}$$	Vasoconstriction, inotropic agents, polycythemia, shock (cardiogenic, hypovolemic), atherosclerosis	Vasodilation, modest hypoxemia, anemic states, drugs (nitrates, milrinone, alpha and calcium channel blockers), shock (septic, anaphylactic, neurogenic)
Mixed venous oxygen saturation (SVO₂)	60–80%		↑O₂ supply: ↑SaO ↑Hgb ↓O₂ demand: ↓VO₂ VO₂, O₂ demand ↓Utilization of O₂ by tissues	↓O₂ supply: ↓CO ↓SaO₂ ↓Hgb ↑O₂ demand: ↑VO₂ ↑CO

(continued)

5

Hemodynamic Parameters (continued)

PARAMETER	NORMAL	FORMULA	CAUSES OF HIGH VALUES	CAUSES OF LOW VALUES
Pulmonary artery occlusive pressure (PAOP) or wedge	8–15 mm Hg		Hypertension, fluid overload, pulmonary hypertension	Dehydration, diuretics, vasodilation
Pulmonary artery pressures (PAP)	15–30 mm Hg (systolic) 8–15 mm Hg (diastolic) 10–20 mm Hg (mean)		Hypertension, vasoconstriction, pulmonary edema, pulmonary hypertension	Dehydration, diuretics (alpha and calcium channel blockers)
Pulmonary vascular resistance index (PVRI)	180–285 dynes/s/ cm^{-5}/m^2	$\dfrac{PAM - PAOP \times 80}{CI}$	Hypoxia, hypercapnia, vasoconstriction, pulmonary edema, pulmonary embolus, COPD, mitral stenosis, shock (cardiogenic, hypovolemic)	Vasodilation, drugs (nitrates, milrinone, alpha and calcium channel blockers), shock (septic, anaphylactic, neurogenic)

Parameter	Normal value	Formula		
Right ventricular pressures (RVP)	15–30 mm Hg (systolic) 2–8 mm Hg (diastolic)		Fluid overload, venous constriction, pulmonary hypertension	Dehydration, diuretic, hemorrhage, venodilation, third spacing, dysrhythmias
Right ventricular stroke work index (RVSWI)	7–12 g/m²/beat	$\dfrac{(PAD - CVP)\,SV}{CI} \times .0136$	Response to catecholamines (beta stimulants, milrinone), normal electrolyte levels, aerobic metabolism, <40% loss of functional myocardium, increased preload	Myocardial infarction, MDF, drugs (beta blockers, calcium channel blockers), hyponatremia, hyperkalemia, anaerobic metabolism, >40% loss of functional myocardium, decreased preload
Stroke volume	60–80 mL/beat	CO/HR	Exercise, bradycardia, positive inotropic agents	Tachycardia, arrhythmias, extreme vasodilation, cardiac tamponade
Systemic vascular resistance index (SVRI)	1970–2390 dynes/s/ cm⁻⁵/m²	$\dfrac{MAP - CVP}{CI} \times 80$	Vasoconstriction, inotropic agents, polycythemia, shock (cardiogenic, hypovolemic), atherosclerosis	Vasodilation, modest hypoxemia, anemic states, drugs (nitrates, milrinone, beta and calcium channel blockers), shock (septic, anaphylactic, neurogenic)

BSA, body surface area; DBP and SBP, diastolic and systolic blood pressure; HR, heart rate; MDF, myocardial depressant factor; PAD, pulmonary artery diastolic pressure; PAM, pulmonary artery (pressure), mean; SaO₂, arterial oxygen saturation.

Cardiac Changes Associated With Aging

ANATOMIC OR PHYSIOLOGIC CHANGE	POTENTIAL CONSEQUENCES
CARDIAC CHANGES	
LV hypertrophy	Decreased LV reserve
	Decreased cardiac output
Cardiac valves thicken and calcify	Increased heart pressures
CONDUCTION CHANGES	
Fibrosis of SA node	Decreased heart rate
	Sick sinus syndrome
Altered baroreceptor reflex	Decreased heart rate
	Orthostatic hypotension
VASCULAR CHANGES	
Elongation and stiffness of aorta	Decreased cardiac output
	Slightly increased BP
Arterial stiffening and thickening	Slightly increased BP

BP, blood pressure; LV, left ventricle; SA, sinoatrial.

Hemodynamic Monitoring Set-Up

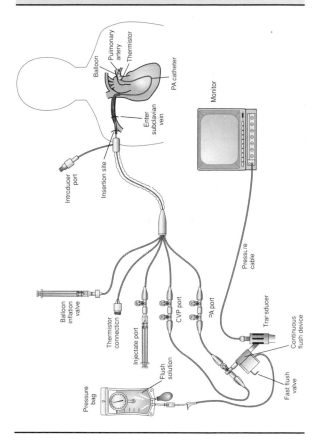

Allen Test

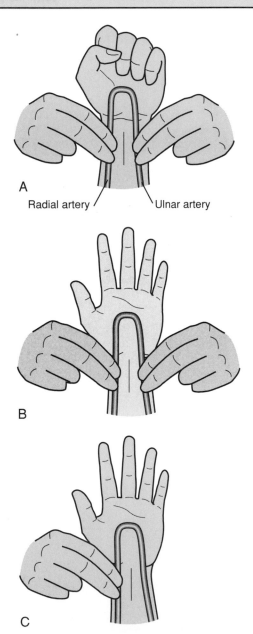

A

Radial artery — — Ulnar artery

B

C

Normal Arterial Waveform

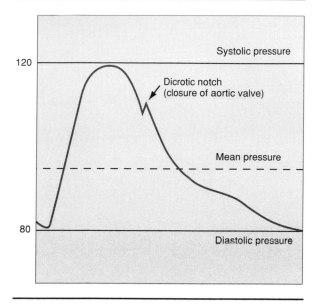

Pulmonary Catheter

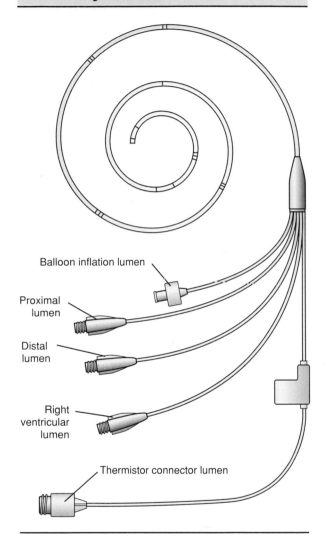

Balloon inflation lumen

Proximal lumen

Distal lumen

Right ventricular lumen

Thermistor connector lumen

Right Atrium Pressure Tracings

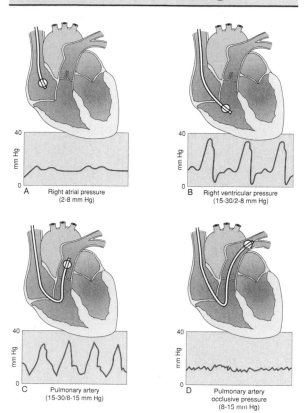

A Right atrial pressure
(2-8 mm Hg)

B Right ventricular pressure
(15-30/2-8 mm Hg)

C Pulmonary artery
(15-30/8-15 mm Hg)

D Pulmonary artery
occlusive pressure
(8-15 mm Hg)

Cardiovascular Assessment

Cardiovascular Risk Factors

MODIFIABLE	NONMODIFIABLE
Cigarette smoking	Age
Hypertension	Gender (male sex)
High LDL-C	Heredity (family history)
Low HDL-C	Race (African-American)
Diabetes mellitus	
Sedentary lifestyle	
Obesity	
Lack of reproductive hormones	
Psychosocial factors	
Type A behavior pattern	
Psychological stress	
Low socioeconomic status	

HDL-C, high-density lipoprotein cholesterol; LDL-C, low-density lipoprotein cholesterol.

Christiana Care—Department of Cardiac Rehabilitation History and Physical Cardiac Risk Factor Inquiry

Name _____
MR # _____

NONMODIFIABLE RISK FACTORS

Family History   ___ MI   ___ CVA   Gender   ___ Female after menopause ___ Age at onset

___ Surgery   ___ HTN   ___ Female not receiving estrogen placement

                                                         ___ Male ___ Male after age 65

MODIFIABLE RISK FACTORS

Hypertension   How long _____ Treatment _____

Diabetes   Type _____ Age at onset _____ Treatment _____

                 Glucose monitoring: Blood _____ Urine _____

                 Frequency _____ HgbA$_1$C _____

                 Patient will bring glucometer to exercise session _____

Tobacco Abuse   Present _____ Past _____

                 Type _____ Amount _____ Method used _____

                 Cessation date _____

                 Reason for cessation _____

                 Interested in a smoking cessation program _____

Hyperlipidemia

Patient is unaware of current cholesterol levels _____

Current levels Date _____ Total _____ HDL _____ LDL _____ Trig _____

Diet AHA/NCEP 1 _____ NCEP 2 _____ Ornish _____ Other _____

ADA _____ Calories _____

Alcohol intake _____ Caffeine intake _____

Would the patient like to meet with the nutritionist while in the program? _____

Obesity

More than 15 lb overweight _____

Current weight _____ Height _____

Patient's desired weight _____ Desired weight loss _____

Stress

Do you currently have any stress that might affect your health? _____

Type A personality _____

Stressors _____

_____

Are you interested in learning more about stress management? _____

Sedentary Lifestyle

Currently compliant with discharge program _____ Able to check pulse _____

Able to resume normal sexual functioning _____

Home exercise equipment or health facility _____

_____

Signature _____ Date _____

Courtesy of the Department of Cardiac Rehabilitation, Christiana Care Health Services, Wilmington, DE.

Risk Stratification Parameters for Monitoring Patients During Exercise

RISK LEVEL	CHARACTERISTICS
Low	Uncomplicated clinical course
	No evidence of myocardial ischemia
	Function capacity > 7 METs
	Normal LV function (EF > 50%)
	Absence of significant ventricular ectopy
Intermediate	ST-segment depression > 2 mm flat or downsloping
	Reversible thallium deficit
	Moderate to good LV function (EF 35–49%)
	Changing or new pattern of angina pectoris
	Failure to comply with exercise intensity prescription
High	Prior MI or infarct involving > 35% of LV
	EF < 35% at rest
	Fall in exercise systolic BP or failure to rise more than 10 mm Hg on exercise tolerance test
	Functional capacity < 5 METs with hypotensive blood pressure response or > 1 mm ST-segment depression
	Congestive heart failure syndrome in hospital
	High-grade ventricular ectopy
	Previous cardiac arrest

BP, blood pressure; EF, ejection fraction; LV, left ventricular; MET, metabolic equivalent; MI, myocardial infarction. Courtesy of the Medical Center of Delaware, Department of Cardiac Rehabilitation.

Guide to Comprehensive Risk Reduction for Patients With Coronary and Other Vascular Disease

RISK INTERVENTION	RECOMMENDATIONS
Smoking Goal complete cessation	Strongly encourage patient and family to stop smoking. Provide counseling, nicotine replacement, and formal cessation programs as appropriate.

Lipid management
Primary goal
LDL <100 mg/dL
Secondary goals
HDL >35 mg/dL;
TG <200 mg/dL

Start AHA Step II Diet in all patients: ≤30% fat, <7% saturated fat, <200 mg/d cholesterol.
Assess fasting lipid profile. In post-MI patients, lipid profile may take 4 to 6 weeks to stabilize. Add drug therapy according to the following guide:

LDL <100 mg/dl	LDL 100 to 130 mg/dL				LDL >130 mg/dL	HDL <35 mg/dL
No drug therapy	Consider adding drug therapy to diet, as follows:				Add drug therapy to diet, as follows:	Emphasize weight management and physical activity. Advise smoking cessation. If needed to achieve LDL goals, consider niacin, statin, fibrate.
	Suggested drug therapy					
	TG <200 mg/dL	TG 200 to 400 mg/dL	TG >400 mg/dL			
	Statin Resin Niacin	Statin Niacin	Consider combined drug therapy (niacin, fibrate, statin)			
	If LDL goal not achieved, consider combination therapy.					

19

Guide to Comprehensive Risk Reduction for Patients With Coronary and Other Vascular Disease (continued)

RISK INTERVENTION	RECOMMENDATIONS
Physical activity <u>Minimum goal</u> 30 minutes 3 to 4 times per week	Assess risk, preferably with exercise test, to guide prescription. Encourage minimum of 30 to 60 minutes of moderate-intensity activity 3 or 4 times weekly (walking, jogging, cycling, or other aerobic activity) supplemented by an increase in daily lifestyle activities (eg, walking breaks at work, using stairs, gardening, household work). Maximum benefit 5 to 6 hours a week. Advise medically supervised programs for moderate- to high-risk patients.
Weight management	Start intensive diet and appropriate physical activity intervention, as outlined above, in patients >120% of ideal weight for height. Particularly emphasize need for weight loss with hypertension, elevated triglycerides, or elevated glucose levels.
Antiplatelet agents/ anticoagulants	Start aspirin 80 to 325 mg/d if not contraindicated. Manage warfarin to international normalized ratio = 2 to 3.5 for post-MI patients not able to take aspirin.
ACE inhibitors post-MI	Start early post-MI in stable high-risk patients (anterior MI, previous MI, Killip class II [S_3 gallop, rales, radiographic CHF]). Continue indefinitely for all with LV dysfunction (ejection fraction ≤40%) or symptoms of failure. Use as needed to manage blood pressure or symptoms in all other patients.

Beta-blockers	Start in high-risk post-MI patients (arrhythmia, LV dysfunction, inducible ischemia) at 5 to 28 days. Continue 6 months minimum. Observe usual contraindications. Use as needed to manage angina rhythm or blood pressure in all other patients.
Estrogens	Consider estrogen replacement in all postmenopausal women. Individualize recommendation consistent with other health risks.
Blood pressure control <u>Goal</u> ≤140/90 mm Hg	Initiate lifestyle modification—weight control, physical activity, alcohol moderation, and moderate sodium restriction—in all patients with blood pressure >140 mm Hg systolic or 90 mm Hg diastolic. Add blood pressure medication, individualized to other patient requirements and characteristics (ie, age, race, need for drugs with specific benefits) **if** blood pressure is not less than 140 mm Hg systolic or 90 mm Hg diastolic in 3 months **or** if *initial* blood pressure is >160 mm Hg systolic or 100 mm Hg diastolic.

ACE indicates angiotensin-converting enzyme; MI, myocardial infarction; TG, triglycerides; LV, left ventricular; CHF, congestive heart failure.

From Smith, S.C., et al. Preventing heart attack and death in patients with coronary disease. Circulation 92:3, 1995. With permission American Heart Association.

Signs and Symptoms of Cardiovascular Disease

SIGNS AND SYMPTOMS	POSSIBLE CARDIAC CAUSE
Dyspnea	Left ventricular failure
	Mitral stenosis
Syncope	Dysrhythmias, especially heart rates >180 and <30
	Aortic stenosis and hypertrophic cardiomyopathy
	Postural hypotension
	Vasovagal reflex
Chest pain or discomfort	Coronary heart disease
	Dissecting aortic aneurysm
	Aortic valve disease
Cyanosis	Congenital heart disease
	Low cardiac output
Dependent edema	Congestive heart failure
Fatigue	Congestive heart failure
	Mitral valve disease
Hemoptysis	Mitral stenosis
Palpitations	Tachydysrhythmias: PSVT, atrial flutter, atrial fibrillation, MAT, VT
	Bradydysrhythmias: Heart block, sinus arrest
	Premature beats

MAT, multifocal atrial tachycardia; PSVT, paroxysmal supraventricular tachycardia; VT, ventricular tachycardia.

Cardiac Palpation and Auscultation Points

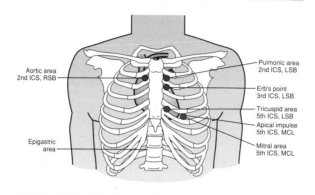

Aortic area
2nd ICS, RSB

Epigastric
area

Pulmonic area
2nd ICS, LSB

Erb's point
3rd ICS, LSB

Tricuspid area
5th ICS, LSB

Apical impulse
5th ICS, MCL

Mitral area
5th ICS, MCL

Grading of Heart Murmurs

Grade	Description
Grade 1 (1/6)	Faint
Grade 2 (2/6)	Quiet
Grade 3 (3/6)	Moderately loud
Grade 4 (4/6)	Loud
Grade 5 (5/6)	Very loud
Grade 6 (6/6)	Heard with stethoscope entirely off chest

Characteristics of Systolic Murmurs*

TYPE	CONDITION/CAUSE	LOCATION	INTENSITY/PITCH	PATTERN/QUALITY	RADIATION
Ejection murmur (midsystolic)	**Aortic stenosis** Forward blood flow through stenotic valve	Second intercostal space, right sternal border	Often loud with a thrill	Crescendo-decrescendo "Diamond-shaped"	Neck →left sternal border → apex
			Medium to high	Often harsh Musical at apex	
	Pulmonic stenosis Forward blood flow through stenotic valve	Second intercostal space, left sternal border	Soft to loud	Crescendo-decrescendo "Diamond-shaped"	Left shoulder and neck
			Medium	Often harsh	

Ejection murmur (holosystolic)						
Ventricular septal defect Blood flow from LV to RV	Left sternal border	Often very loud with a thrill	High	Plateau S_1 —— S_2 Often harsh		Wide
Mitral regurgitation Backflow of blood into left atrium	Apex	Soft to loud	Medium to high	Plateau S_1 —— S_2 Blowing		Left axilla
Tricuspid regurgitation Backflow of blood into right atrium	Left lower sternal border	Variable	Medium	Plateau S_1 —— S_2 Blowing		Right of sternum, xiphoid area

*Systolic murmurs occur between S_1 and S_2 in the following valve positions: aortic/pulmonic → open; mitral/tricuspid → closed.

Characteristics of Diastolic Murmurs*

TYPE	CONDITION/CAUSE	LOCATION	INTENSITY/PITCH	PATTERN/QUALITY	RADIATION
Ejection murmur	**Mitral stenosis** Forward blood flow through stenotic valve	Apex	Grade 1–4 Low	Decrescendo–crescendo Rumbling	Little to none
Regurgitant murmur	**Aortic regurgitation** Backflow of blood into ventricle	Second to fourth left intercostal space	Grade 1–3 High	Early decrescendo Blowing	Apex, right sternal border

*Common diastolic murmurs occur between S_2 and S_1 in the following valve positions: aortic pulmonic → closed; mitral/tricuspid → open.

Pulse Amplitude Documentation

0 = Absent
1 = Diminished
2 = Normal
3 = Increased
4 = Bounding

Cardiovascular Laboratory and Diagnostic Tests

Normal Serum Electrolyte, Blood
  Urea Nitrogen, and Creatinine
  Values

Normal Serum Hemoglobin
  and Hematocrit Values

Goals for Blood Cholesterol
  and Lipid Levels

Patterns of Cardiac Enzymes in Acute
  Myocardial Infarction

Recommended Therapeutic Range
  for Oral Anticoagulation

Contraindications to Magnetic
  Resonance Imaging

Nursing Care of the Patient
  Undergoing Transesophageal
  Echocardiography

Indications for Cardiac Catheterization

Normal Hemodynamic Parameters
  Obtained from Cardiac
  Catheterization

Contraindications to Cardiac
  Catheterization

Complications of Cardiac
  Catheterization

Atrial Fibrillation Criteria

Atrial Fibrillation Electrocardiogram Strip

Junctional Rhythm Criteria

Junctional Rhythm Electrocardiogram Strip

Junctional Tachycardia Criteria

Junctional Tachycardia Electrocardiogram Strip

Premature Junctional Complex Criteria

Premature Junctional Complex Electrocardiogram Strip

First-Degree Atrioventricular Block Criteria

First-Degree Atrioventricular Block Electrocardiogram Strip

Second-Degree Atrioventricular Block, Mobitz Type I Criteria

Second-Degree Atrioventricular Block, Mobitz Type I Electrocardiogram Strip

Second-Degree Atrioventricular Block, Mobitz Type II Criteria

Second-Degree Atrioventricular Block, Mobitz Type II Electrocardiogram Strip

Third-Degree Atrioventricular Block Criteria

Third-Degree Atrioventricular Block Electrocardiogram Strip

Premature Ventricular Complex Criteria

Premature Ventricular Complex Electrocardiogram Strip

Ventricular Tachycardia Criteria

Normal Serum Electrolyte, Blood Urea Nitrogen, and Creatinine Values

COMPONENT	NORMAL RANGE
Sodium	135–145 mEq/L
Potassium	3.5–5.0 mEq/L
Calcium, total	8.5–10.5 mg/dL
Calcium, ionized	4.5–5.1 mg/dL
Magnesium	1.5–2.5 mg/dL
Blood urea nitrogen (BUN)	6–20 mg/dL
Creatinine	0.8–1.2 mg/dL
BUN-to-creatinine ratio	10:1

Normal Serum Hemoglobin and Hematocrit Values*

	HEMOGLOBIN	HEMATOCRIT
Adult male	14.0–17.4 g/dL	42–52%
Adult female	12.0–16.0 g/dL	36–48%

*Values vary with age and race.

Goals for Blood Cholesterol and Lipid Levels*

Total cholesterol	<200 mg/dL
Low-density lipoprotein (LDL)	<130 mg/dL
High-density lipoprotein (HDL)	>35 mg/dL
Triglycerides	<200 mg/dL
Cholesterol-to-HDL ratio	<4 mg/dL

*Although the reference range for values of cholesterol and lipids varies according to sex and age, the recommended target goals (for adults) are the same regardless of age, race, or sex.

Patterns of Cardiac Enzymes in Acute Myocardial Infarction

ENZYME	EARLIEST RISE	PEAK	NORMALIZATION
CK	4–6 hours	12–24 hours	3–4 days
CK-MB	4–6 hours	12–24 hours	2–3 hours
LDH	12–24 hours	3–6 days	7–10 days
Troponin I	3–7 hours	14–18 hours	5–7 days

CK, creatine kinase; CK-MB, creatine kinase–myocardial bands; LDH, lactate dehydrogenase.

Recommended Therapeutic Range for Oral Anticoagulation

INDICATION	INTERNATIONAL NORMALIZED RATIO (INR)
Primary and secondary prevention of venous thrombosis	
Treatment of pulmonary embolism	
Prevention of systemic embolism	2.0–3.0
Tissue heart valves	
Post myocardial infarction	
Valvular heart disease	
Atrial fibrillation	
Mechanical prosthetic valves	2.5–3.5

Adapted from Hirsh J, Dalen J, Deykin D, et al: Oral anticoagulants: Mechanism of action, clinical effectiveness and optimal therapeutic range. Chest 108:231S, 1995.

Contraindications to Magnetic Resonance Imaging

Absolute

- Implanted cardiac pacemakers and implanted cardiac defibrillators; MRI may cause device to shut down, fire, or function inappropriately owing to the strong magnetic field
- Epicardial pacemaker wires
- Implanted drug infusion pumps
- Cochlear (inner ear) implants
- Metal vascular or aneurysm clips, especially cerebral
- Metal artificial heart valve
- Certain intrauterine devices

Potential (Patient Should Be Assessed by a Radiologist)

- Artificial joint replacements
- Dental braces and bridges
- Surgical wires and clips from previous procedures
- Metal meshes and plates
- Other foreign objects in the body
- Pregnancy

Nursing Care of the Patient Undergoing Transesophageal Echocardiography

Before the Procedure

- Assess for contraindications: history of esophageal dysfunction, cancer, strictures, or surgery
- History of adverse reactions to anesthetics or sedatives
- Explain the procedure to the patient
- Obtain a signed informed consent
- Patient to have nothing by mouth for at least 4–6 hours prior to the procedure
- Intravenous line or heparin lock should be inserted
- Dentures or oral prosthesis removed
- Patient should void before procedure

- Suction set-up should be in place and functioning
- Resuscitation equipment available
- Patient placed on the cardiac monitor and pulse oximeter

During the Procedure

- Throat may be sprayed with topical anesthetic, which may cause a bitter taste and the sensation of a swollen tongue
- Patient positioned on left side with head flat or slightly elevated
- Patient positioned in "chin to chest" position to allow for better passage of the endoscope through the oropharynx
- Continuous, conscious sedation
- Suction as needed
- Inform the patient of progress and provide reassurance
- Continuous monitoring of blood pressure, heart rate, and oxygenation

After the Procedure

- Patient should sit up or be positioned on side
- Encourage patient to cough
- Patient should receive nothing by mouth until the gag reflex enables him or her to protect the airway (30 minutes to several hours)
- Give lozenges; sore throat possible for a couple days
- If procedure was done as outpatient, instruct patient not to drive for the next 12 hours if sedation was given during the procedure; best to have someone drive the patient home
- Instruct patient to call the physician in the event of hemoptysis, pain, or dyspnea

Indications for Cardiac Catheterization

1. Suspected or known coronary artery disease
   a. New-onset angina
   b. Unstable angina
   c. Evaluation before a major surgical procedure
   d. Silent ischemia
   e. Positive exercise treadmill test
   f. Atypical chest pain or coronary spasm
2. Acute myocardial infarction (AMI)
   a. Unstable angina after infarction
   b. Failed thrombolytic therapy
   c. Cardiogenic shock secondary to AMI
   d. Mechanical complications secondary to AMI (e.g., ventricular septal defect, rupture of ventricular wall, papillary muscle)
3. Sudden cardiovascular death
4. Valvular heart disease
5. Congenital heart disease (before anticipated corrective surgery)
6. Aortic dissection
7. Pericardial constriction or tamponade
8. Cardiomyopathy
9. Initial and follow-up assessment for heart transplant

From Kern MJ, et al. (eds): The Cardiac Catheterization Handbook, 2nd ed. St. Louis, Mosby–Year Book, 1994, p 3.

Normal Hemodynamic Parameters Obtained From Cardiac Catheterization

CHAMBER OR VESSEL	PRESSURE READING (mm Hg)
Right atrium	2–8 (mean)
Right ventricle	15–30 (systolic)
	2–8 (diastolic)
Pulmonary artery	15–30 (systolic)
	4–12 (diastolic)
Pulmonary artery: occlusive pressure	4–12 (mean)
Left atrium	4–12 (mean)
Left ventricle	100–140 (systolic)
	4–12 (diastolic)
Aorta	100–140 (systolic)
	60–90 (diastolic)
	70–90 (mean)
Cardiac output	4–8 L/minute
Cardiac index	2.5–4.0 L/minute

Contraindications to Cardiac Catheterization

Absolute Contraindication

- Inadequate equipment, personnel, or catheterization facility

Relative Contraindications

- Uncontrolled congestive heart failure, hypertension, dysrhythmias
- Recent cerebral vascular accident (< 1 month)
- Infection or fever
- Electrolyte imbalance
- Acute gastrointestinal bleeding or anemia
- Pregnancy
- Anticoagulation (or known, uncontrolled bleeding diathesis)
- Uncooperative patient
- Medication intoxication (e.g., digoxin)
- Renal failure

From Kern MJ, et al. (eds): The Cardiac Catheterization Handbook, 2nd ed. St. Louis, Mosby–Year Book, 1994, p 4.

Complications of Cardiac Catheterization

Death ($<0.2\%$)
Myocardial infarction ($<0.5\%$)
Cerebral vascular accident ($<0.5\%$)
Serious dysrhythmia ($<1.0\%$)
- Ventricular tachycardia
- Ventricular fibrillation
- Atrial fibrillation
- Supraventricular tachydysrhythmia
- Heart block asystole

Vascular injury ($<1.0\%$)
- Hemorrhage (local, retroperitoneal, pelvic)
- Pseudoaneurysm
- Thrombosis, embolism, or air embolism
- Aortic dissection

Cardiac perforation, tamponade
Contrast reaction, anaphylaxis, or nephrotoxicity
Protamine reaction
Infection
Congestive heart failure
Vasovagal reaction

From Kern MJ, et al. (eds): The Cardiac Catheterization Handbook, 2nd ed. St. Louis, Mosby–Year Book, 1994, p 4.

Information for Patients Undergoing Cardiac Catheterization

The purpose of cardiac catheterization is to evaluate the function of your heart and its blood flow. Before the procedure

- Do not eat or drink anything 6 hours prior to the test
- If you are allergic to any medications or x-ray dye, inform your physician prior to the test
- Inform your physician of all medications you are currently taking. If you are taking a medicine called warfarin (Coumadin), a blood thinner, your physician will instruct you when to stop taking this medicine prior to the test

During the procedure

- You will be placed on a narrow table
- Cardiac catheterization should not be painful; let your physician or nurse know if you are uncomfortable during the procedure
- One side of your groin (or one arm) will be shaved, and sterile drapes will be placed to keep the area as clean as possible; do not touch these drapes
- After giving you a local numbing medicine in your groin (or arm), your physician will then place a catheter (similar to an intravenous line) into your groin (or arm)
- It will be very important for you to cough and hold your breath when you are asked to do so
- Inform the staff if you have any chest pain or discomfort
- A large camera will rotate around you and take pictures of your heart as the physician injects dye into your coronary arteries and heart. The dye will make you feel very hot for a few seconds, and you may experience some chest pain

After the procedure

- Your physician will be able to tell you the results of your test shortly after the catheterization. Together, you will be able to plan what to do if you are found to have heart disease
- After the procedure, the catheter(s) will be removed from your groin (or arm), and pressure will be held on the area for about 30 minutes to prevent bleeding. You must lie flat for 4 to 8 hours, as directed
- During the recovery period, your vital signs, the dressing, and the pulses in your feet will be checked frequently. It is very important to maintain bedrest as you are instructed
- After the catheterization, you will be encouraged to drink as many fluids as possible to help flush the dye out of your body through the kidneys

---

Adapted from Ricciuti CG (ed): Cardiac Diagnostic Tests: A Guide for Nurses. Philadelphia, W.B. Saunders, 1997, p 289.

Electrocardiographic Waves and Intervals of the Normal Cardiac Cycle

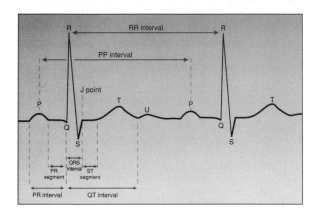

Normal R-Wave Progression of the Precordial Leads

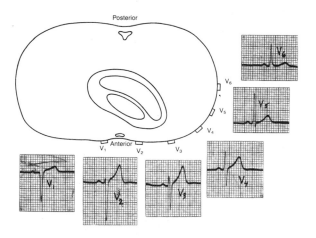

From Phillips R, Feeney M: The Cardiac Rhythms, 3rd ed. Philadelphia, W.B. Saunders, 1990.

A, Proper Lead Positioning for Modified Chest Lead 1 and Modified Chest Lead 6; B, Proper Lead Positioning for Lead V₁ with Five-Lead Bedside Monitor

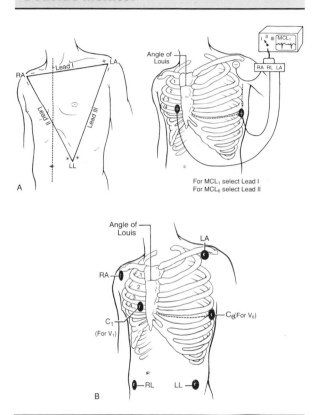

For MCL₁ select Lead I
For MCL₆ select Lead II

From Drew BJ: Bedside electrocardiogram monitoring. AACN Clin Issues Crit Care Nurs 4(1):26, 28, 1993.

Recommended Leads for Cardiac Monitoring

For Monitors With Five-Lead Patient Cables

First choice
  Single-lead monitoring: V_1
  Dual-lead monitoring: V_1 plus the limb lead appropriate for clinical situation
Second choice
  Substitute V_6 for V_1 when patient cannot have electrode at sternal border
  or
  When QRS amplitude is not adequate for optimized computerized dysrhythmia monitoring

For Monitors With Three-Lead Patient Cables

First choice
  MCL_1
Second choice
  MCL_6

Tips for selecting a limb lead appropriate for the patient's clinical situation

1. Atrial flutter: II, III, or aVF
2. Inferior MI: II, III, or aVF (pick lead with maximum ST-segment elevation on 12-lead ECG)
3. Anterior MI: pick lead with maximum ST-segment elevation on 12-lead ECG
4. Following angioplasty: III or aVF (whichever has the tallest R wave)
5. If three channels are available for ECG monitoring, the combination of V_1 + I + aVF has the following advantages:
    a. Best dysrhythmia lead = V_1
    b. Atrial flutter = aVF
    c. Inferior MI or postangioplasty = aVF
    d. Axis determination = I and aVF

ECG, electrocardiogram; MCL, modified chest lead; MI, myocardial infarction.
Adapted from Drew BJ: Bedside electrocardiogram monitoring. AACN Clinical Issues in Critical Care Nursing 4(1):25–33, 1993.

Normal Sinus Rhythm Criteria

ECG Criteria

- Rate: 60–100 beats/minute
- Rhythm: regular; RR and PP intervals are constant
- P wave: normal and upright in lead II; P wave precedes each QRS complex
- PR interval: 0.12–0.20 seconds and constant
- QRS complex: 0.04–0.12 seconds

Normal Sinus Rhythm Electrocardiogram Strip

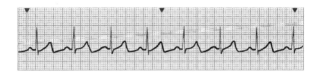

From Cohn E, Gilroy-Doohan M: Flip & See ECG. Philadelphia, W.B. Saunders, 1996, p 71.

Sinus Bradycardia Criteria

ECG Criteria

- Rate: 40–60 beats/minute
- Rhythm: regular to slightly irregular
- P wave: normal and upright in lead II; one P wave precedes each QRS complex
- PR interval: 0.12–0.20 seconds and constant
- QRS complex: 0.04–0.12 seconds

Cause

- Increased vagal stimulation
- Medical conditions: atherosclerotic heart disease, myocardial infarction, hypothermia, increased intracranial pressure, hypoendocrine states (e.g., Addison's disease, myxedema coma)

(continued)

Sinus Bradycardia Criteria (continued)

- Medications: digoxin, calcium channel blockers, beta blockers, central nervous system depressants (e.g., morphine, sedatives)

Treatment

Usually no treatment is indicated; patients who do demonstrate signs and symptoms of low cardiac output and hemodynamic compromise (e.g., hypotension, changes in level of consciousness, angina, syncope) may require one or more of the following:

- Identification and treatment of the underlying cause of the bradycardia
- Atropine
- Isoproterenol (Isuprel)
- Pacemaker: transcutaneous, temporary, and/or permanent
- Advanced Cardiac Life Support (ACLS): Bradycardia Algorithm

Sinus Bradycardia Electrocardiogram Strip

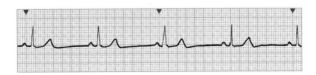

From Cohn E, Gilroy-Doohan M: Flip & See ECG. Philadelphia, W.B. Saunders, 1996, p 75.

Sinus Tachycardia Criteria

ECG Criteria

- Rate: 100–160 beats/minute
- Rhythm: regular to slightly irregular
- P wave: normal and upright in lead II; one P wave precedes each QRS complex; P waves are sometimes not visible at higher heart rates but can usually be found on 12-lead ECG
- PR interval: 0.12–0.20 seconds and constant
- QRS complex: 0.04–0.12 seconds

Cause

- Enhanced automaticity
- Caffeine-containing products, i.e., coffee, tea, chocolate
- Medical conditions: anxiety, pain, fever, hypotension, anemia, myocardial infarction, shock, congestive heart failure
- Medications: dopamine (Intropin), aminophylline, epinephrine (Adrenalin)

Treatment

- Determine and treat the underlying cause (e.g., fever, pain, hypovolemia)
- Cardiac medications: beta blockers, calcium channel blockers
- Central nervous system depressants: antianxiety agents, tranquilizers, pain medication
- ACLS: Tachycardia Algorithm

Sinus Tachycardia Electrocardiogram Strip

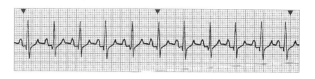

From Cohn E, Gilroy-Doohan M: Flip & See ECG. Philadelphia, W.B. Saunders, 1996, p 77.

Sinus Dysrhythmia Criteria

ECG Criteria

- Rate: 40–100 beats/minute; periods of slower and faster heart rates may alternate
- Rhythm: irregular RR intervals with corresponding changes in the rate
- P wave: normal and upright in lead II; one P wave precedes each QRS complex
- PR interval: 0.12–0.20 seconds and may vary slightly
- QRS complex: 0.04–0.12 seconds

Cause

- Respiratory variation most common etiology

Treatment

- None required

Sinus Dysrhythmia Electrocardiogram Strip

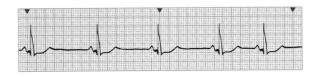

From Cohn E, Gilroy-Doohan M: Flip & See ECG. Philadelphia, W.B. Saunders, 1996, p 73.

Sinus Arrest Criteria

ECG Criteria

- Rate: 60–100 beats/minute, often <60 beats/minute due to missed beats
- Rhythm: irregular RR intervals; rhythm is characterized by missed or dropped beats; rhythm remains regular before and after missed beats
- P wave: one P wave precedes each QRS complex; absent during missed beat
- PR interval: normal
- QRS complex: normal

Cause

- Cardiac origin: cardiomyopathy, rheumatic heart disease, myocardial infarction
- See Sinus Bradycardia Criteria

Treatment

- No treatment necessary in asymptomatic patients
- Reduce or eliminate any medications that may be contributing to the cause
- Temporary pacing may be necessary in symptomatic patients
- If SA node is unable to restore normal pacing, a permanent pacemaker may be indicated
- ACLS: Bradycardia Algorithm

Sinus Arrest Electrocardiogram Strip

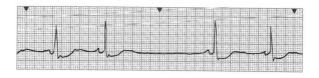

Premature Atrial Contraction Criteria

ECG Criteria

- Rate: variable; usually 60–100 beats/minute
- Rhythm: irregular; when PACs occur, the pause after the PAC is *not* usually compensatory; the sinus beat after the PAC does not occur at normal time because the SA node timing is interrupted
- P waves: premature P wave with possible abnormal configuration (flat, slurred, notched, inverted, diphasic, or wide) or lost in T wave or QRS complex of sinus beat; P wave of the sinus beat is normal
- PR interval: sinus beat: normal; PAC: varies depending on site of ectopic pacemaker
- QRS complex: usually normal

Cause

- Stimulants: catecholamines, caffeine, nicotine, excessive alcohol consumption
- Cardiac disease: myocardial infarction, CHF
- Electrolyte disturbances: hypokalemia, hypermetabolic states
- Medical conditions: hypoxemia, chronic obstructive pulmonary disease
- Emotions: anxiety, fear
- Medications: central nervous system stimulants, digoxin, over-the-counter medications containing stimulants

Treatment

- Usually no treatment needed; continue to monitor
- Treat underlying cause (e.g., decrease consumption of caffeine, correct hypoxemia)
- Consider electrolyte imbalance, digoxin toxicity, early warning of CHF

Premature Atrial Contraction Electrocardiogram Strip

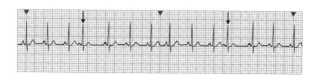

From Cohn E, Gilroy-Doohan M: Flip & See ECG. Philadelphia, W.B. Saunders, 1996, p 79.

Paroxysmal Atrial Tachycardia Criteria

ECG Criteria

- Rate: atrial rate is between 150 and 250 beats/minute; onset is usually sudden and often initiated by a premature atrial contraction
- Rhythm: regular or slightly irregular
- P waves: ectopic P waves with possible abnormal contour; may be difficult to see in any of the 12 leads
- PR interval: <0.12 seconds; may be difficult to see or measure
- QRS complex: usually normal

Cause

- See Premature Atrial Contraction Criteria

Treatment

- Often self-limiting
- Treatment is aimed at correcting underlying cause
- Vagal nerve stimulation (e.g., carotid sinus massage, Valsalva maneuvers) may possibly slow rate
- Consider adenosine, beta blockers, calcium channel blockers, digoxin to slow rate
- Consider cardioversion if hemodynamically unstable (e.g., angina, hypotension, changes in level of consciousness)
- ACLS: Tachycardia Algorithm, Electrical Cardioversion Algorithm

Paroxysmal Atrial Tachycardia Electrocardiogram Strip

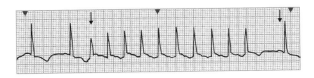

Phillips R, Feeney M: The Cardiac Rhythms, 3rd ed. Philadelphia, W.B. Saunders, 1990, p 154.

Atrial Flutter Criteria

ECG Criteria

- Rate: atrial: between 250 and 350 beats/minute; ventricular rate: depends on degree of AV block; varying degrees of AV conduction or block may be present in ratios of 2:1, 3:1, 4:1
- Rhythm: atrial: usually regular (PP intervals constant) but can be irregular due to varying conduction ratios; ventricular: usually regular (RR intervals are constant) but can be irregular due to varying conduction ratios
- AV conduction: depends on rate and degree of AV block
- P waves: "sawtooth" flutter waves; usually peaked, uniform in width
- PR interval: not usually measurable
- QRS complex: usually narrow

Cause

- Rarely occurs in the absence of organic heart disease: coronary artery disease, cardiomyopathy, congestive heart failure, valvular heart disease
- Medical conditions: pulmonary disease, chronic obstructive pulmonary disease, pulmonary embolism

Treatment

- Treatment is aimed at the restoration of normal sinus rhythm
- Consider: digoxin, propranolol, quinidine, diltiazem, verapamil to slow ventricular rate

- Consider cardioversion if hemodynamically unstable (e.g., angina, hypotension, changes in level of consciousness)
- ACLS: Tachycardia Algorithm, Electrical Cardioversion Algorithm

Atrial Flutter Electrocardiogram Strip

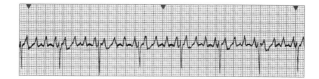

Atrial Fibrillation Criteria

ECG Criteria

- Rate: atrial: between 350 and 600 beats/minute; ventricular: range from 100–180 beats/minute depending on AV conduction
- Rhythm: ventricular: irregular and usually rapid depending on degree of AV block
- AV conduction: ventricles respond irregularly to excessive impulses from atria
- P waves: no visible P waves; fibrillating, wavelike, erratic baseline of varying shapes and sizes
- PR interval: not visible or measurable
- QRS complex: usually narrow unless conduction is delayed through the ventricles

Cause

- Associated with underlying cardiac disease (e.g., coronary artery disease, valvular heart disease) and extracardiac disease (e.g., chronic obstructive pulmonary disease, pulmonary embolism, thyroid disorders)
- See also Premature Atrial Contraction Criteria

(continued)

Atrial Fibrillation Criteria (continued)

Treatment

- Treatment aimed at controlling the ventricular response and the restoration of sinus rhythm
- Consideration of digoxin, quinidine, beta blockers, calcium channel blockers to slow ventricular rate and/or to convert to normal sinus rhythm
- Cardioversion if patient hemodynamically unstable (e.g., angina, hypotension, changes in level of consciousness)
- ACLS: Tachycardia Algorithm, Electrical Cardioversion Algorithm

Atrial Fibrillation Electrocardiogram Strip

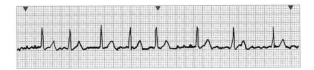

Note irregular RR interval. From Cohn E, Gilroy-Doohan M: Flip & See ECG. Philadelphia, W.B. Saunders, 1996, p 85.

Junctional Rhythm Criteria

ECG Criteria

- Rate: 40–60 beats/minute
- Rhythm: usually regular; may be slightly irregular
- P waves: P wave may precede QRS complex; may be lost in QRS complex and not visible; may follow the QRS complex (retrograde conduction); may be upright in leads I, aVR, and aVL and inverted in leads II, III, and aVF
- PR interval: if P wave precedes QRS complex, the PR interval is usually short (< 0.12 seconds)
- QRS complex: usually normal

Cause

- Coronary artery disease, congestive heart failure, cardiomyopathy, rheumatic heart disease, myocardial infarction, electrolyte imbalances
- Sinus dysrhythmias: sinus bradycardia, sinus arrest
- Medications: beta blockers, calcium channel blockers, digoxin, central nervous system depressants

Treatment

- Treatment aimed at eliminating underlying cause
- Treatment required is similar to treatment for symptomatic sinus bradycardia: may require atropine, isoproterenol to increase ventricular rate; may require temporary or permanent pacemaker when patient is symptomatic (e.g., hypotensive)
- ACLS: Bradycardia Algorithm

Junctional Rhythm Electrocardiogram Strip

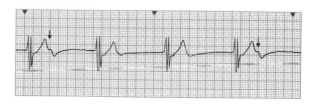

Junctional Tachycardia Criteria

ECG Criteria

- Rate: accelerated: 60–100 beats/minute; junctional tachycardia: 100–180 beats/minute; paroxysmal junctional tachycardia: 180–250 beats/minute
- Rhythm: usually regular, may be slightly irregular
- P waves: P wave may precede QRS complex; may be hidden in the QRS complex; may follow the QRS complex (retrograde conduction); upright in leads I, aVR, aVL and inverted in leads II, III, aVF
- PR interval: if P wave precedes QRS complex, PR interval is usually short (<0.12 seconds)
- QRS complex: usually normal

Cause

- See Junctional Rhythm Criteria

Treatment

- Identify and treat underlying cause (e.g., digitalis toxicity, acute myocardial infarction, electrolyte disturbances)
- Consider vagal maneuvers (carotid sinus massage, Valsalva maneuvers)
- Consideration of medications useful to treat atrial tachycardias (e.g., calcium channel blockers, digoxin, central nervous system depressants)
- ACLS: Tachycardia Algorithm

Junctional Tachycardia Electrocardiogram Strip

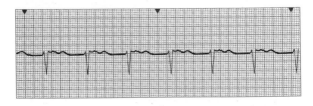

Premature Junctional Complex Criteria

ECG Criteria

- Rate: usually normal; dependent on rate of underlying rhythm
- Rhythm: usually irregular due to premature beat
- P waves: P wave of the premature junctional complex (PJC) may come before, during, or after the QRS complex; usually upright in leads I, aVR, and aVL; inverted in leads II, III, and aVF
- PR interval: if P wave of the PJC precedes the QRS complex, the PR interval is usually short (<0.12 seconds)
- QRS complex: usually normal

Cause

- Can occur in healthy individuals without a history of heart disease
- Coronary artery disease, congestive heart failure, cardiomyopathy, rheumatic heart disease, myocardial infarction
- Excessive caffeine, alcohol, tobacco consumption

Treatment

- Treatment aimed at eliminating underlying cause

Premature Junctional Complex Electrocardiogram Strip

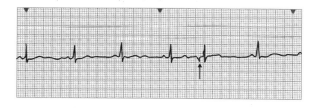

First-Degree Atrioventricular Block Criteria

ECG Criteria

- Rate: 60–100 beats/minute
- Rhythm: regular, RR intervals are constant
- AV conduction: prolonged
- P wave: normal and upright in lead II; one P wave precedes each QRS complex
- PR interval: >0.20 seconds and constant
- QRS complex: 0.04–0.12 seconds

Cause

- Can be a normal variant
- Associated with initial degenerative disease of the conduction system
- Coronary artery disease, myocarditis, myocardial infarction
- Medications: beta blockers, calcium channel blockers, digitalis toxicity

Treatment

- Usually none; continue to monitor
- Consider modifying or eliminating causative medication, if appropriate

First-Degree Atrioventricular Block Electrocardiogram Strip

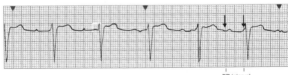

PR interval
.40 sec

Second-Degree Atrioventricular Block, Mobitz Type I Criteria

ECG Criteria

- Rate: atrial: 60–100 beats/minute; ventricular: slower than atrial rate; depends on ratio of P waves to QRS complexes
- Rhythm: atrial: regular; ventricular: irregular, RR interval becomes progressively shorter, group beating usually occurs leading to a *regularly irregular* rhythm
- AV conduction: some impulses from the SA node do not conduct through to the ventricles; AV conduction ratios are usually constant
- PR interval: becomes progressively longer with each cycle until a dropped beat occurs (P wave present but lacks a succeeding QRS)
- QRS complex: usually normal

Cause

- Almost always associated with some type of heart disease (e.g., myocardial infarction, coronary artery disease)
- See First-Degree Atrioventricular Block Criteria

Treatment

- Often no treatment necessary; observation; continue to monitor
- Identify underlying cause and treat (e.g., drug toxicity, myocardial infarction)
- Consider atropine, temporary pacemaker if patient is symptomatic (e.g., angina, hypotension, changes in level of consciousness)
- ACLS: Bradycardia Algorithm

Second-Degree Atrioventricular Block, Mobitz Type I Electrocardiogram Strip

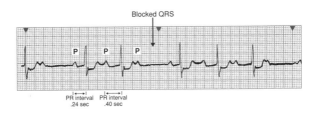

Blocked QRS

PR interval .24 sec   PR interval .40 sec

Second-Degree Atrioventricular Block, Mobitz Type II Criteria

ECG Criteria

- Rate: see Mobitz type I
- Rhythm: atrial: regular; ventricular: regular or irregular depending on the block
- AV conduction: some impulses do not conduct through to the ventricles; AV conduction ratios are usually constant
- P wave: more P waves than QRS complexes
- PR interval: constant; may be prolonged (>0.20 seconds)
- QRS complex: periodically "dropped" after a P wave; normal duration if block is at level of bundle of His, >0.12 seconds if bundle branch block present

Cause

- See First-Degree Atrioventricular Block Criteria
- Usually associated with cardiac disease

Treatment

- Treatment aimed at preventing progression to third-degree AV block
- Identify underlying cause and treat (e.g., drug toxicity, myocardial infarction)
- Consideration of atropine, isoproterenol to increase ventricular rate

- Consideration of dopamine in the setting of hypotension
- Temporary transvenous pacemaker if patient is symptomatic (e.g., hypotension, angina, changes in level of consciousness)
- ACLS: Bradycardia Algorithm

Second-Degree Atrioventricular Block, Mobitz Type II Electrocardiogram Strip

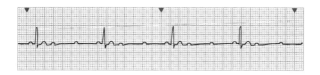

From Cohn E, Gilroy-Doohan M: Flip & See ECG. Philadelphia, W.B. Saunders, 1996, p 101.

Third-Degree Atrioventricular Block Criteria

ECG Criteria

- Rate: atrial: 60–100 beats/minute; ventricular: 20–60 beats/minute
- Rhythm: atrial and ventricular rates are regular but independent of each other
- AV conduction: no atrial impulses are conducted to the ventricles; ventricular conduction is ectopic
- P waves: normal but are *not* related to QRS complexes and some may be hidden in the QRS complexes
- PR interval: varies
- QRS complex: normal if impulse originated in AV junction; wide (>0.12 seconds) if originating in ventricles

Cause

- Coronary artery disease, congestive heart failure, myocardial infarction
- Medications: beta blockers, calcium channel blockers, digitalis toxicity

(continued)

Third-Degree Atrioventricular Block Criteria (continued)

Treatment

- Identify underlying cause; most patients will be symptomatic (e.g., dizziness, hypotension, angina, changes in level of consciousness) and require urgent treatment
- Atropine, isoproterenol, dopamine
- Temporary or permanent transvenous pacing may be necessary
- ACLS: Bradycardia Algorithm

Third-Degree Atrioventricular Block Electrocardiogram Strip

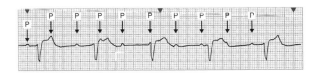

From Cohn E, Gilroy-Doohan M: Flip & See ECG. Philadelphia, W.B. Saunders, 1996, p 103.

Premature Ventricular Complex Criteria

ECG Criteria

- Rate and rhythm: determined by underlying rhythm
- P wave: P waves are usually not visible in the premature ventricular complex (PVC); if present, may occur before, during (hidden in), or after the ectopic beat
- PR interval: determined by the underlying rhythm
- QRS complex: PVC: wide (>0.12 seconds), bizarre, distorted; T wave of PVC deflects in opposite direction (polarity) of QRS complex; may be unifocal or multifocal; compensatory pause follows PVC

Cause

- Coronary artery disease, myocardial infarction, congestive heart failure, conduction system disease
- Electrolyte imbalances: hypokalemia, hypermetabolic states
- Anxiety, fear, stress
- Caffeine, excessive use of alcohol or nicotine
- Medications: epinephrine, dopamine, aminophylline
- May occur in individuals without a history of heart disease

Treatment

- Consideration of treatment with frequent PVCs (>5–6/ minute), bigeminy, trigeminy, multifocal PVCs
- Treatment aimed at determining and managing the underlying cause (e.g., electrolyte imbalance, myocardial infarction, congestive heart failure)
- Administer lidocaine (LidoPen), procainamide (Pronestyl), bretylium (Bretylol), as needed

Premature Ventricular Complex Electrocardiogram Strip

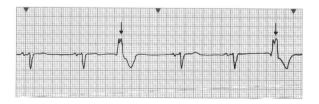

Ventricular Tachycardia Criteria

ECG Criteria

- Rate: ventricular: 150–250 beats/minute
- Rhythm: ventricular: regular or slightly irregular
- Conduction: originating in ventricles
- P waves: usually hidden in QRS complex
- PR interval: not visible and not measurable
- QRS complex: wide and bizarre; similar to PVCs

Cause

- See Premature Ventricular Complex Criteria
- Coronary artery disease, congestive heart failure, myocardial infarction, cardiomyopathy
- Electrolyte imbalances, hypermetabolic states
- Medications: digoxin, quinidine, central nervous system stimulants, thyroid medications

Treatment

- Treatment depends on severity and duration of the dysrhythmia and patient's response to the rhythm (asymptomatic versus symptomatic)
- Sustained ventricular tachycardia is considered a medical emergency—immediate intervention is required
- Investigate and correct underlying electrolyte imbalance (e.g., hypokalemia)
- Medications: lidocaine, bretylium, procainamide
- Electrical cardioversion is necessary for hemodynamically unstable ventricular tachycardia or when patient is not responsive to drug therapy
- ACLS: Tachycardia Algorithm, Ventricular Fibrillation/Pulseless Ventricular Tachycardia Algorithm, Electrical Cardioversion Algorithm
- Torsades de pointes: remove offending drug, magnesium sulfate, overdrive pacing
- Implantable cardiodefibrillator for long-term prophylaxis

Ventricular Tachycardia Electrocardiogram Strip

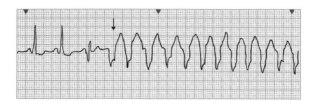

Ventricular Fibrillation Criteria

ECG Criteria

- Rate: rapid, chaotic; too rapid to count
- Rhythm: irregular and chaotic; ventricular rhythm lacks pattern
- Conduction: no organized conduction
- P waves: none
- PR interval: none
- QRS complex: none; undulating, fibrillating baseline

Cause

- See Ventricular Tachycardia Criteria

Treatment

- Ventricular fibrillation is considered a medical emergency—immediate intervention is required
- Immediate direct-current defibrillation
- Immediate cardiopulmonary resuscitation
- ACLS: Ventricular Fibrillation/Pulseless Ventricular Tachycardia Algorithm

Ventricular Fibrillation Electrocardiogram Strip

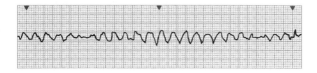

From Cohn E, Gilroy-Doohan M: Flip & See ECG. Philadelphia, W.B. Saunders, 1996, p 91.

Asystole Criteria

ECG Criteria

- Rate: no atrial or ventricular activity
- Rhythm: none; either a straight, flat line or fine, chaotic, and incomprehensible tracing
- Conduction: no atrial or ventricular activity
- P wave: none
- PR interval: none
- QRS complex: none; either a straight, flat line or fine, chaotic, and incomprehensible tracing

Treatment

- Immediate cardiopulmonary resuscitation
- Distinction necessary from fine ventricular fibrillation, check in two leads
- ACLS: Asystole Treatment Algorithm

Asystole Electrocardiogram Strip

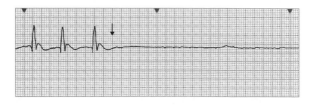

Electrocardiogram Summary of Right Bundle Branch Block and Left Bundle Branch Block

Right Bundle Branch Block (RBBB)

1. Wide QRS complex (>0.12 seconds)
2. Triphasic rsR^1 in MCL_1/V_1; triphasic qRs in MCL_6/V_6
3. ST segment and T wave slope away from the major deflection (i.e., negative in MCL_1/V_1 and positive in MCL_6/V_6)
4. If the QRS complex has the typical RBBB contour but measures 0.09–0.011 seconds, the diagnosis of incomplete RBBB is made

Left Bundle Branch Block (LBBB)

1. Wide QRS complex (>0.12 seconds)
2. Large Q in MCL_1/V_1 (about one third of LBBBs have an initial little r wave in these leads, which is not well understood, but it results in an rS complex with the S wave prolonged and large amplitude); a large R wave in MCL_6/V_6
3. ST segment and T wave slope away from the dominant wave of the QRS
4. Widened QRS complexes with LBBB contour measuring 0.10–0.12 seconds are all called incomplete LBBB or left intraventricular conduction delay

Morphology of Right Bundle Branch Block in Precordial Leads V_1–V_6

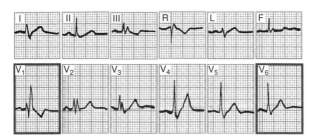

Morphology of Left Bundle Branch Block in Precordial Leads V_1–V_6

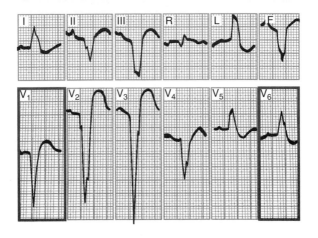

ST-Segment and T-Wave Changes Associated With (A) Myocardial Ischemia, (B) Injury, and (C) Necrosis

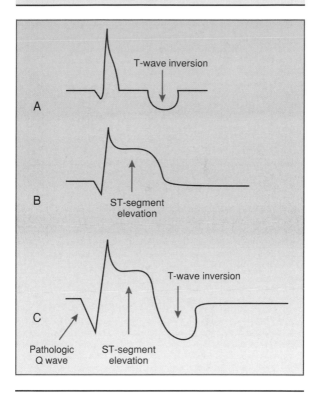

Common Electrocardiogram Changes With Myocardial Infarction Over Time

TYPE OF INFARCTION	ECG CHANGES
Acute infarction	ST-segment elevation hyperacute, coved, and often marked Q waves are small or absent Hyperacute or tall, peaked T waves Reciprocal ST-segment depression often present
Recent infarction	Pathologic Q waves ST-segment elevation minimal or absent T wave inversion often present and possibly marked Reciprocal ST-segment depression minimal or absent
Old infarction	Q waves present ST-segment elevation absent T-wave inversion minimal or absent No reciprocal ST-segment changes

Indications for the Implantation of a Permanent Cardiac Pacemaker

DISORDER	CLASS OF INDICATION
Sinus node dysfunction	I. Sinus node dysfunction with documented symptomatic bradycardia
	II. Sinus node dysfunction with heart rates < 40 beats/minute; no clear association between symptoms and bradycardia
	III. No symptoms
AV block	I. Symptomatic complete or second-degree AV block with heart rates ≤ 40 beats/minute, or consequence of His bundle ablation
	II. Asymptomatic second-degree type II or complete heart block with heart rates > 40 beats/minute
	III. First-degree AV block or asymptomatic type I AV block
Bifascicular or trifascicular	I. Fascicular block with intermittent complete heart block associated with symptoms or second-degree type II AV block with or without symptoms
	II. HV intervals > 100 msec or fascicular block associated with syncope that cannot be ascribed to other causes
	III. Asymptomatic fascicular block or fascicular block with associated first-degree AV block
Neurogenic syncope	I. Recurrent syncope provoked by carotid sinus stimulation; pauses of > 3 seconds induced by minimal carotid sinus pressure
	II. Syncope associated with bradycardia reproduced by head-up tilting
	III. Recurrent syncope in the absence of a cardioinhibitory response
Cardiomyopathy	I. None
	II. Severely symptomatic patients with hypertrophic cardiomyopathy refractory to drug therapy (may become class I in the future)
	III. Severely symptomatic patients with dilated cardiomyopathy (may become class II in the future)

AV, atrioventricular; HV interval, the conduction interval between the His bundle and the ventricular myocardium. From Kusumoto FM, Goldschlager N: Cardiac pacing. N Engl J Med 334(2):90, 1996.

Coronary Artery Disease

Types of Angina

TYPE	DESCRIPTION
Acute coronary insufficiency	Angina that is changing or unstable, often increasing in intensity and duration; this angina can lead to a myocardial infarction if left untreated
Angina decubitus	Angina associated with lying in the recumbent position
Crescendo angina	Angina that is increasing with frequency with less intense precipitating factors
Nocturnal angina	Angina that has its onset associated with the REM (rapid eye movement) phase of sleep
Preinfarction angina	Unstable angina that progresses into a myocardial infarction
Prinzmetal's angina (variant)	Angina associated with the vasospasm of one or more of the coronary arteries; it is often severe and not induced by effort; it may occur at or around the same time of the day; it may or may not occur in the presence of atherosclerosis
Progressive angina	Angina that is newly diagnosed and increasing in severity
Stable (chronic) angina	Angina that has not changed in intensity, duration, or frequency for at least 2 months; often exercise or exertion induced; can be mild or severe
Unstable (acute) angina	Angina that is changing or unstable, often increasing in intensity and duration; this angina can lead to a myocardial infarction if left untreated

Using the P, Q, R, S, and T Acronym to Assess Angina

P: Precipitating factors	Emotional upset Exercise or exertion Eating a large meal Temperature extremes Sexual intercourse
Q: Quality of discomfort	Substernal or left-sided pain, pressure Burning, throbbing, or stabbing pain Heaviness like "an elephant sitting on chest" Tightness like "a vise around chest" Shortness of breath "Worse pain ever experienced"
R: Region of discomfort	Substernal or left-sided chest pain Radiating down left arm Intrascapular Radiating into jaw and neck Epigastric Numbness or tingling in left arm Left shoulder, left axillary region Can be any combination of the above
S: Severity	Use a scale from 0–10, with 10 representing the worse pain ever experienced by the patient; a subjective scale helps clinicians to determine the patient's perception of pain as well as the effects of interventions
T: Time	Investigate the frequency and duration of attacks: When did the chest pain start? Stop? What did the patient do before seeking help and did it work?

Differential Diagnosis of Angina-Like Discomfort

CONDITION	RELATED SYMPTOMATOLOGY
Angina	Increasing episodes, ECG changes, presence of atherosclerosis
Costochondriasis	Chest wall pain due to inflammation that increases in quality on palpation of area
Myocardial infarction	Acute ECG changes, lasting longer than 15 minutes
Pericarditis	Sharp, stabbing pain aggravated by deep breathing, rotating chest, or supine position; relieved by sitting up and leaning forward; presence of pericardial friction rub
Dissecting aortic aneurysm	Anterior chest pain, radiating to thoracic area of back or abdominal pain; described as tearing pain; lower blood pressure in one arm, absent pulses, murmur in aortic region
Mitral valve prolapse syndrome	Substernal stabbing pain that may radiate to left arm, back, jaw; variable palpitations, dizziness, or dyspnea
Pulmonary hypertension	Substernal pain, aggravated by effort; pain usually associated with dyspnea, right ventricular lift
Spontaneous pneumothorax	Unilateral pain; sharp, well localized; painful breathing; dyspnea, cough, fever, dull to flat percussion; occasional pleural rub
Gastrointestinal disorders	Lower substernal area, epigastric, right or left quadrant burning, colic-like, aching pain; precipitated by meals or lying down; nausea, regurgitation, food intolerance

Medications Used in the Treatment of Coronary Artery Disease

MEDICATION	MECHANISM OF ACTION
Aspirin	Inhibition of platelet aggregation; antiinflammatory agent
Heparin	Prevention of thrombus propagation
Nitrates	
Nitroglycerin (sublingual)	Peripheral and coronary vasodilation
Nitroglycerin (IV)	Peripheral and coronary vasodilation
Analgesics (IV)	
Morphine sulfate (IV)	Analgesia, anxiolysis, vasodilation
Meperidine (IV)	Analgesia, anxiolysis, vasodilation
Beta blockers	
Propranolol	Reduction of oxygen consumption by reducing cardiac contractility; decreases sinoatrial and atrioventricular node velocity and reduction in blood pressure
Metoprolol	Same as above
Calcium channel blockers	
Diltiazem	Coronary and peripheral vasodilation; reduces afterload, heart rate, and contractility
ACE inhibitors	
Captopril, enalapril, lisinopril, quinapril	Vasodilation, reduction in afterload
Cardiac glycosides	
Digoxin	Increases cardiac output, decreases sinoatrial and atrioventricular conduction, and reduces oxygen consumption
Antidysrhythmias	Restore normal heart rhythm
Lidocaine, procainamide, adenosine, beta blockers, calcium channel blockers, digoxin	

PTCA/INTERVENTION ALGORITHM

	PRE INTERVENTION DATE: ___	POST INTERVENTION DATE: ___
ASSESSMENTS & CONSULTS	CT SURGEON STANDBY	
LABS, DIAGNOSTICS & INTERVENTIONS	CBC, CHEM 7, TYPE & HOLD, PTT, ACT SHAVE & PREP BILATERAL GROINS INTERVENTION CARE PER STANDARD*	PTT & WITH HEPARIN CHANGES, ACT 4H POST AND TILL BASELINE WITH SHEATH PULL NEXT DAY: CK, H&H IF STENT: ACT'S PER STANDARD INTERVENTION CARE PER STANDARD* D/C SHEATH BEDREST X 48 HOURS IF STENT GROIN CARE*
MEDICATIONS & IV'S	HOLD MEDS FOR INTERVENTION AS ORDERED PRE INTERVENTION MEDS* IV ACCESS*	RESUME MEDS POST SHEATH REMOVAL D/C HEPARIN PRE SHEATH PULL
DIET & ACTIVITY	NPO POST MIDNIGHT	RESUME DIET OOB TO CHAIR AND AMBULATE PER INTERVENTION & SHEATH PULL STANDARDS*
TEACHING & FOLLOW-UP	INSTRUCTIONS & CONSENT	GROIN CARE* POST INTERVENTION INSTRUCTIONS*

NURSING CARE PERFORMED
 	
KEY: *NSG Activities
V = Variance
N = No Var.
	Δ 1. V ____
	  N ____
	Δ 2. V ____
	  N ____
	Δ 3. V ____
	  N ____
		Δ 1. V ____
		  N ____
		Δ 2. V ____
		  N ____
		Δ 3. V ____
		  N ____

NSG/AMI;OTC Rev. 4/95
This pathway was developed as a guideline only. It is not intended to be used as a substitute for clinical judgment. Acceptable medical practice generally does include a variety of responses to a particular problem.

5

Acute Myocardial Infarction

Acute Myocardial Infarction: ECG Evidence, Associated Coronary Arteries, and Potential Complications

Area of Infarct	ECG EVIDENCE		Associated Coronary Artery	Potential Complications
	Leads Reflecting Infarct Area Directly	Leads Reflecting Reciprocal Changes		
LEFT VENTRICLE				
Lateral wall, high	I, aVL	II, III, aVF	Left circumflex	Pump failure, conduction disturbances
Inferior wall	II, III, aVF	I, aVL, V_5, V_6	Right coronary, possibly left circumflex	Sinoatrial and atrioventricular nodal conduction disturbances; valve dysfunction
Septal wall	V_1–V_2	II, III, aVF	Left anterior descending	Pump failure, conduction disturbances

Anterior wall	V_2–V_4	II, III, aVF	Left anterior descending	Pump failure, conduction disturbance
Lateral wall, low (apical area)	V_5–V_6	II, III, aVF	Left anterior descending	Pump failure, conduction disturbance
Posterior	V_7–V_9*	V_1–V_3	Posterior descending, right coronary, or left circumflex	Atrioventricular nodal conduction disturbance
RIGHT VENTRICLE†				
	V_4R	—	Right coronary	Atrioventricular nodal conduction disturbance, valve dysfunction, hypotension

*Leads are placed on the left posterior chest wall at the fifth intercostal space, beginning at the left posterior axillary line.

†Right ventricular infarction is present in approximately one third of patients with inferior myocardial infarctions, and assessment of this lead should be routinely performed in all patients diagnosed with an acute inferior myocardial infarction.

Clinical Presentation of Acute Myocardial Infarction

SYSTEM	POSSIBLE FINDINGS
Neurologic **Patients >85 years**	Restlessness Acute confusion* Syncope* Stroke*

Cardiovascular	Chest pain
	ECG findings:
	    Bradycardia
	    Tachycardia
	    Ventricular ectopy
	    Atrioventricular blocks
	Normotension or hypotension
	S_3 or S_4
	Systolic murmur
	Decreased cardiac output:
	    Diminished capillary refill
	    Diminished peripheral pulses
	Jugular venous distention
	Peripheral edema

Respiratory **African-American males** **Patients >85 years** **Women**	Shortness of breath* Orthopnea Tachypnea Crackles Frothy sputum
Integumentary	Diaphoresis
Gastrointestinal **Female patients**	Pallor Nausea* Vomiting*
Genitourinary	Diminished urine output
Psychosocial	Anxiety Agitation Anger Denial

*Indicates physical findings that are often the primary presenting symptoms for these populations but may also be associated symptoms for anyone experiencing acute myocardial infarction.

Comparison of Major Thrombolytic Agents

FEATURE	DRUG		
	Streptokinase	Recombinant Tissue Plasminogen Activator*	Anisoylated Plasminogen Streptokinase Activator
Dose	1.5 million IU in 60 min (750,000 IU over first 10 min)	100 mg in 90 min (15 mg over 1–2 min, then 50 mg over next 30 min, then 35 mg over next 60 min)	30 U in 2–5 min
Route	IV	IV†	IV‡
Peak effect	1–2 hours	20–120 min	45 min
Duration of effect	Up to 12 hr	Up to 3 hr	4–6 hr
Elimination (half-life)	Biphasic: initially, 18 min; subsequent, 83 min	Rapid, > 80% cleared within 10 min	90–120 min

*Accelerated dosage schedule for patients >67 kg.

†Should be administered through a dedicated intravenous (IV) line, using a volumetric infusion pump. After infusion, IV line should be flushed with 25–30 mL of normal saline solution.

‡Directly into vein or via free flowing IV line of normal saline solution.

Monitoring a Patient on Bleeding Precautions for Complications

LABORATORY DATA	PHYSICAL ASSESSMENT DATA	SUBJECTIVE DATA
Reduction in hemoglobin, hematocrit	Ecchymosis, petechiae Bleeding gums	Anxiety Palpitations
Coagulation studies exceeding therapeutic goals (aPTT, ACT)	Gross blood in stool, urine, emesis, nasogastric drainage, sputum	
Reduced platelets	Bleeding from intravenous sites, previous venipuncture or intramuscular injection sites	
Occult blood in stool, urine, emesis, nasogastric drainage, sputum	Changes in mentation, level of consciousness Changes in vital signs: decreased blood pressure, increased heart rate Cool, clammy skin	

ACT, activated clotting time; aPTT, activated partial thromboplastin time.

Pharmacotherapeutic Adjuncts and Nursing Considerations for a Patient Experiencing an Acute Myocardial Infarction

DRUG	RECOMMENDED DOSE	GENERAL NURSING CONSIDERATIONS
NITRATES		
Nitroglycerin (NTG) Sublingual (SL) Translingual (TL) Intravenous (IV)	0.4 µg every 5 min × 3 1 spray (0.4 mg) every 5 min × 3 Begin at 5–10 µg/min and titrate (5–10 µg/min every 5–10 min) until pain is relieved or patient becomes hypotensive (systolic pressure <90 mm Hg); maximum dose not established	Monitor effectiveness of drug by assessing patient for chest pain using standardized pain scale For IV, SL, TL routes, monitor BP every 5 minutes until stable; for other routes, monitor BP per orders and assess for orthostatic hypotension Consider interactive effects on BP if administered with other hypotensive agents Administer acetaminophen if headache develops Monitor for S/S of methemoglobinemia* (pallor, dyspnea, cyanosis, coma) with prolonged use of high doses of IV NTG Use infusion pump to deliver IV NTG Dilute drug in compatible solution and use glass or nonabsorbable container; use non-PVC administration sets (to limit absorption of drug by tubing)
When tapering IV NTG, consider conversion to: Oral	2.5 mg TID–QID to maximum of 26 mg/day	
Topical	1–2 inches every 8 hours to maximum of 5 inches every 3–6 hours	

(continued)

83

Pharmacotherapeutic Adjuncts and Nursing Considerations for Patients Experiencing an Acute Myocardial Infarction (continued)

DRUG	RECOMMENDED DOSE	GENERAL NURSING CONSIDERATIONS
NITRATES (continued)		
When tapering IV NTG, consider conversion to: Transdermal	0.2–0.4 mg/hr for 10–12 hr/day to maximum of 0.8 mg/hr for 10–12 hr/day	When tapering IV NTG, reduce dose gradually to limit rebound chest pain and/or hypertension
ANTIPLATELETS		
Aspirin (ASA)	80–160 mg/day	Administer with meals to limit gastrointestinal distress
If unable to tolerate ASA:		Consider interactive effects on risk for bleeding if administered with other anticoagulants
Ticlopidine hydrochloride	250 mg BID	Therapeutic response for ticlopidine hydrochloride may take 2–3 mo to achieve
ANTICOAGULANT		
Heparin	80 U/kg IV bolus, then 18 U/kg/hr infusion to keep aPTT 1.5–2.0 times the patient control	Initiate bleeding precautions per policy In case of severe bleeding, administer protamine sulfate to neutralize heparin

		Monitor for interactive effects: NTG decreases anticoagulant effect; ASA increases anticoagulant effect
		Monitor for S/S of heparin-induced thrombocytopenia† (HIT or white clot syndrome): impaired peripheral perfusion, pulmonary embolism, AMI, stroke)
		Use infusion pump to deliver dose

ANALGESICS

Morphine	2–5 mg IV every 5–15 min	Administer dose slowly and observe for drop in BP, respiratory rate, central nervous system effects (sedation, confusion)
If RVMI, consider meperidine	10–50 mg every 2–4 hr	Consider interactive effects on BP when administered with other hypotensive drugs
		Assess the effectiveness of drug in relieving chest pain by using standardized pain scale
		Severe hypotensive effects most likely when dose is administered rapidly
		Administer naloxone (Narcan) for S/S of severe hypotension and/or respiratory depression
		Consider reduced dose in elderly patients and in those with hepatic or renal impairment

(continued)

Pharmacotherapeutic Adjuncts and Nursing Considerations for Patients Experiencing an Acute Myocardial Infarction (continued)

DRUG	RECOMMENDED DOSE	GENERAL NURSING CONSIDERATIONS
BETA BLOCKERS		
Metoprolol	5 mg IV every 5 minutes × 3, then 50 mg PO 15 min after completion of IV dosing; repeat PO dose every 6 hr for 48 hr	Administer IV dose slowly and monitor patient for symptomatic bradycardia, hypotension, and S/S of CHF and heart block Monitor for interactive effects: increase in lidocaine levels; may mask hypoglycemic symptoms in patients taking antidiabetic agents; additive effect on BP in patients receiving other hypotensive medication
Atenolol	5 mg IV every 5 minutes × 2, then 50 mg PO at 10 min after completion of IV dosing; repeat PO dose every 12 hr for 7 days	Consider reduced dose in elderly patients and in those with hepatic (metoprolol) and renal (atenolol) impairment Abrupt cessation of drug may precipitate chest pain, ventricular dysrhythmias, or acute myocardial infarction
ACE INHIBITORS		
Captopril	6.25 mg PO as a test dose, then titrate to 50 mg TID	Assess BP and heart rate at 1 to 2 hr (peak effect) after administering test dose Severe allergic reactions include angioedema and stridor Monitor patient for symptomatic hypotension, orthostatic hypotension

Monitor for interactive effects: increase in serum digoxin levels, additive effects on BP in patients receiving other hypotensive medication

Consider reduced dose in elderly patients and in those with renal impairment; may see hyperkalemia in patients with renal insufficiency and hypoglycemia in patients with diabetes

Administer 1 hour before or 2 hours after meals

Abrupt cessation of drug can precipitate hypertension

ANTIDYSRHYTHMIC

Lidocaine

Bolus dose of 1.0–1.5 mg/kg, may repeat dose (0.5 mg/kg) every 5–10 min not to exceed a total dose of 3 mg/kg
Initiate maintenance infusion of 2–4 mg/min

Monitor ECG for effectiveness in controlling ventricular ectopy; may cause worsening of dysrhythmias

Assess blood pressure every 5 min during loading dose and every 15–60 min once stable

Use lower bolus doses in the elderly and in patients with liver disease and CHF

Assess for adverse central nervous system effects (tremors, confusion, and agitation) and S/S of toxicity (somnolence, seizures, respiratory depression, hypotension, cardiac arrest); rapid injection is often associated with seizures

Monitor for interactive effects: increased risk for hypotension, bradycardia, and toxicity when administered with beta blockers

Monitor serum lidocaine levels

Use infusion pump to deliver continuous dose

(continued)

Pharmacotherapeutic Adjuncts and Nursing Considerations for Patients Experiencing an Acute Myocardial Infarction (continued)

DRUG	RECOMMENDED DOSE	GENERAL NURSING CONSIDERATIONS
OTHERS		
Magnesium	1–4 g IV bolus over 5–20 min, then 0.5–1.0 g/hr × 24 hr	Rapid injection may cause hypotension, heart block, or cardiac arrest Monitor vital signs every 15 min after bolus dose Assess respiratory status: rate, rhythm, quality Monitor for S/S of hypermagnesemia (loss of deep tendon reflexes, fatal respiratory paralysis) Treat toxicity with calcium gluconate to reverse respiratory depression and heart block Titrate as needed and based on appropriate laboratory or assessment data Discontinue once patient's condition stabilizes
Oxygen	2–4 L/min via nasal cannula	

AMI, acute myocardial infarction; BP, blood pressure; HIT, heparin-induced thrombocytopenia; PVC, polyvinyl chloride; RVMI, right ventricular myocardial infarction; S/S, signs and symptoms.

*Methemoglobinemia is a rare side effect that results from the oxidation of the heme iron by nitrates to the ferric state (methemoglobin), making it incapable of transporting oxygen.

†HIT is found in approximately 10% of patients receiving heparin therapy and is thought to be a result of the production of antiplatelet antibodies that induce clotting.

Heparin Dosing Nomograms

| WEIGHT-BASED DOSES | | NON–WEIGHT-BASED DOSES | |
| Initial dose: 80 U/kg bolus, then 18 U/kg/hr | | Initial dose: 5000 U bolus, then 1000 U/hr | |
aPTT* (sec)	Dosage Adjustment	aPTT* (sec)	Dosage Adjustment
<35 (<1.2 × control)	80 U/kg bolus, increase maintenance dose by 4 U/kg/hr	<35 (<1.2 × control)	5000 U bolus, increase maintenance dose by 200 U/hr
35–45 (1.2– 1.5 × control)	40 U/kg bolus, increase maintenance dose by 2 U/kg/hr	35–45 (1.2– 1.5 × control)	2500 U bolus, increase maintenance dose by 100 U/hr
46–70 (1.5– 2.3 × control)	No change	46–70 (1.5– 2.3 × control)	No change
71–90 (2.3– 3 × control)	Decrease maintenance dose by 2 U/kg/hr	71–90 (2.3– 3 × control)	Decrease maintenance dose by 100 U/hr
>90 (>3 × contro.)	Hold infusion for 1 hour, then decrease maintenance dose by 3 U/kg/hr	>90 (>3 × control)	Hold infusion for 1 hour, then decrease maintenance dose by 200 U/hr

aPTT, activated partial thromboplastin time.

*Drawn 6 hours after initial dose and every 6 hours after dosage adjustment.

From Bowlby H, Hisle K, Clifton GD: Heparin as adjunctive therapy to coronary thrombolysis in acute myocardial infarction. Heart Lung 24(4):299, 1995.

Absolute Contraindications to Thrombolysis

Active or recent (4 weeks) internal bleeding
Intracranial neoplasm or recent head trauma
Prolonged, traumatic cardiopulmonary resuscitation
Suspected aortic dissection
History of hemorrhagic cerebrovascular accident
Sustained systemic blood pressure over 200/120 mm
    Hg despite medication
Trauma or surgery that is a potential bleeding source
    in the past 4 weeks

From Morris DC: Treatment of acute myocardial infarction by invasive cardiology techniques. Semin Thorac Cardiovasc Surg 7:184–190, 1995.

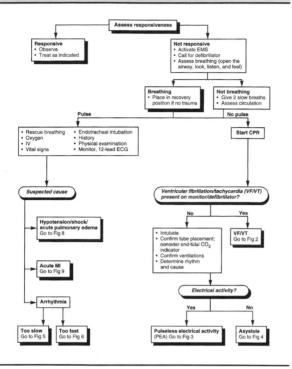

Universal Algorithm for Adult Emergency Cardiac Care

ACC/AHA Figure 1
From the American Heart Association. *Advanced Cardiac Life Support,* © American Heart Association, 1997.

Automated External Defibrillation Treatment Algorithm: Emergency Cardiac Care Pending Arrival of ACLS Personnel

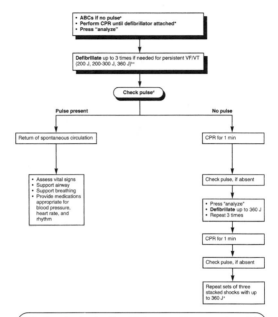

- ABCs if no pulse*
- Perform CPR until defibrillator attached*
- Press "analyze"

⬇

Defibrillate up to 3 times if needed for persistent VF/VT (200 J, 200-300 J, 360 J)ᵇᶜ

⬇

Check pulse*

Pulse present ← → **No pulse**

Pulse present:
Return of spontaneous circulation
⬇
- Assess vital signs
- Support airway
- Support breathing
- Provide medications appropriate for blood pressure, heart rate, and rhythm

No pulse:
CPR for 1 min
⬇
Check pulse, if absent
⬇
- Press "analyze"
- **Defibrillate** up to 360 J
- Repeat 3 times
⬇
CPR for 1 min
⬇
Check pulse, if absent
⬇
Repeat sets of three stacked shocks with up to 360 Jᵉ

*Health professionals with a duty to respond to a person in cardiac arrest should have a defibrillator available immediately or within 1-2 min.

a. The single rescuer with an AED should verify unresponsiveness, open the airway (A), give two respirations (B), and check the pulse (C). If a full cardiac arrest is confirmed, the rescuer should attach the AED and proceed with the algorithm.

b. Pulse checks not required after shocks 1,2,4, and 5 unless "no shock indicated" message is displayed.

c. If no shock is indicated, check pulse, repeat 1 min of CPR, check pulse again, and then reanalyze. After three "no shock indicated" messages, repeat "analyze" period every 1-2 min.

d. For hypothermic patients limit shocks to 3. See hypothermia algorithm.

e. If VF persists after 9 shocks, repeat sets of three stacked shocks with 1 min of CPR between each set until no "shock indicated" message is received. Shock until VF is no longer present or the patient converts to a perfusing rhythm.

ACC/AHA Figure 2A
From the American Heart Association. *Advanced Cardiac Life Support,* © American Heart Association, 1997.

Ventricular Fibrillation/Pulseless Ventricular: Tachycardia Algorithm

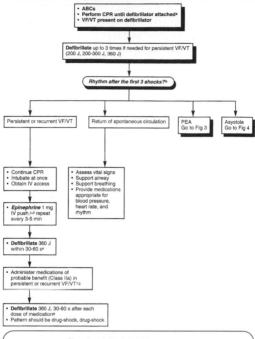

- ABCs
- Perform CPR until defibrillator attached[a]
- VF/VT present on defibrillator

↓

Defibrillate up to 3 times if needed for persistent VF/VT
(200 J, 200-300 J, 360 J)

↓

Rhythm after the first 3 shocks?[b]

Persistent or recurrent VF/VT | Return of spontaneous circulation | PEA Go to Fig 3 | Asystole Go to Fig 4

Persistent or recurrent VF/VT:
- Continue CPR
- Intubate at once
- Obtain IV access

↓

- **Epinephrine** 1 mg IV push,[c,d] repeat every 3-5 min

↓

- **Defibrillate** 360 J within 30-60 s[e]

↓

- Administer medications of probable benefit (Class IIa) in persistent or recurrent VF/VT[f,g]

↓

- **Defibrillate** 360 J, 30-60 s after each dose of medication[e]
- Pattern should be drug-shock, drug-shock

Return of spontaneous circulation:
- Assess vital signs
- Support airway
- Support breathing
- Provide medications appropriate for blood pressure, heart rate, and rhythm

---

Class I: definitely helpful
Class IIa: acceptable, probably helpful
Class IIb: acceptable, possibly helpful
Class III: not indicated, may be harmful

a. Precordial thump is a Class IIb action in witnessed arrest, no pulse, and no defibrillator immediately available.

b. Hypothermic cardiac arrest is treated differently after this point. *See hypothermia algorithm.*

c. The recommended dose of **epinephrine** is 1 mg IV push every 3-5 min. If this approach fails, several Class IIb dosing regimens can be considered:
   - Intermediate: **epinephrine** 2-5 mg IV push, every 3-5 min
   - Escalating: **epinephrine** 1 mg-3 mg-5 mg IV push, 3 min apart
   - High: **epinephrine** 0.1 mg/kg IV push, every 3-5 min

d. **Sodium bicarbonate** 1 mEq/kg is Class I if patient has known preexisting hyperkalemia.

e. Multiple sequenced shocks are acceptable here (Class I), especially when medications are delayed.

f. Medication sequence:
   - **Lidocaine** 1.0-1.5 mg/kg IV push. Consider repeat in 3-5 min to maximum dose of 3 mg/kg. A single dose of 1.5 mg/kg in cardiac arrest is acceptable.
   - **Bretylium** 5 mg/kg IV push. Repeat in 5 min at 10 mg/kg.
   - **Magnesium sulfate** 1-2 g IV in torsades de pointes or suspected hypomagnesemic state or refractory VF.
   - **Procainamide** 30 mg/min in refractory VF (maximum total 17 mg/kg).

g. **Sodium bicarbonate** 1 mEq/kg IV:
   Class IIa
   - If known preexisting bicarbonate-responsive acidosis
   - If overdose with tricyclic antidepressants
   - To alkalinize the urine in drug overdoses
   Class IIb
   - If intubated and continued long arrest interval
   - Upon return of spontaneous circulation after long arrest interval
   Class III
   - Hypoxic lactic acidosis

ACC/AHA Figure 2
From the American Heart Association. *Advanced Cardiac Life Support,* © American Heart Association, 1997.

Pulseless Electrical Activity Algorithm: (Electromechanical Dissociation)

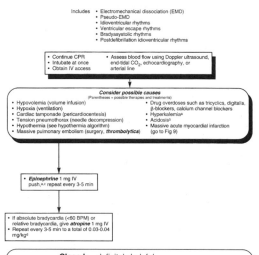

Includes
- Electromechanical dissociation (EMD)
- Pseudo-EMD
- Idioventricular rhythms
- Ventricular escape rhythms
- Bradyasystolic rhythms
- Postdefibrillation idioventricular rhythms

- Continue CPR
- Intubate at once
- Obtain IV access

- Assess blood flow using Doppler ultrasound, end-tidal CO_2, echocardiography, or arterial line

Consider possible causes
(Parentheses = probable therapies and treatments)

- Hypovolemia (volume infusion)
- Hypoxia (ventilation)
- Cardiac tamponade (pericardiocentesis)
- Tension pneumothorax (needle decompression)
- Hypothermia (see hypothermia algorithm)
- Massive pulmonary embolism (surgery, **thrombolytics**)
- Drug overdoses such as tricyclics, digitalis, β-blockers, calcium channel blockers
- Hyperkalemia[a]
- Acidosis[b]
- Massive acute myocardial infarction (go to Fig 9)

- **Epinephrine** 1 mg IV push,[a,c] repeat every 3-5 min

- If absolute bradycardia (<60 BPM) or relative bradycardia, give **atropine** 1 mg IV
- Repeat every 3-5 min to a total of 0.03-0.04 mg/kg[d]

Class I: definitely helpful
Class IIa: acceptable, probably helpful
Class IIb: acceptable, possibly helpful
Class III: not indicated, may be harmful

a. **Sodium bicarbonate** 1 mEq/kg is Class I if patient has known preexisting hyperkalemia.

b. **Sodium bicarbonate** 1 mEq/kg:
   Class IIa
   - If known preexisting bicarbonate-responsive acidosis
   - If overdose with tricyclic antidepressants
   - To alkalinize the urine in drug overdoses
   Class IIb
   - If intubated and continued long arrest interval
   - Upon return of spontaneous circulation after long arrest interval
   Class III
   - Hypoxic lactic acidosis

c. The recommended dose of **epinephrine** is 1 mg IV push every 3-5 min. If this approach fails, several Class IIb dosing regimens can be considered:
   - Intermediate: **epinephrine** 2-5 mg IV push, every 3-5 min
   - Escalating: **epinephrine** 1 mg-3 mg-5 mg IV push, 3 min apart
   - High: **epinephrine** 0.1 mg/kg IV push, every 3-5 min

d. The shorter **atropine** dosing interval (3 min) is possibly helpful in cardiac arrest (Class IIb).

ACC/AHA Figure 3
From the American Heart Association. *Advanced Cardiac Life Support,* © American Heart Association, 1997.

Asystole Treatment Algorithm

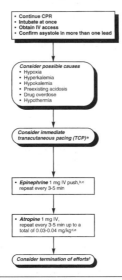

- Continue CPR
- Intubate at once
- Obtain IV access
- Confirm asystole in more than one lead

Consider possible causes
- Hypoxia
- Hyperkalemia
- Hypokalemia
- Preexisting acidosis
- Drug overdose
- Hypothermia

Consider immediate transcutaneous pacing (TCP)[a]

- *Epinephrine* 1 mg IV push,[b,c] repeat every 3-5 min

- *Atropine* 1 mg IV, repeat every 3-5 min up to a total of 0.03-0.04 mg/kg[d,e]

Consider termination of efforts[f]

Class I: definitely helpful
Class IIa: acceptable, probably helpful
Class IIb: acceptable, possibly helpful
Class III: not indicated, may be harmful

a. TCP is a Class IIb intervention. Lack of success may be due to delays in pacing. To be effective TCP must be performed early, simultaneously with drugs. Evidence does not support routine use of TCP for asystole.

b. The recommended dose of ***epinephrine*** is 1 mg IV push every 3-5 min. If this approach fails, several Class IIb dosing regimens can be considered:

- Intermediate: ***epinephrine*** 2-5 mg IV push, every 3-5 min
- Escalating: ***epinephrine*** 1 mg-3 mg-5 mg IV push, 3 min apart
- High: ***epinephrine*** 0.1 mg/kg IV push, every 3-5 min

c. ***Sodium bicarbonate*** 1 mEq/kq is Class I if patient has known preexisting hyperkalemia.

d. The shorter ***atropine*** dosing interval (3 min) is Class IIb in asystolic arrest.

e. ***Sodium bicarbonate*** 1 mEq/kg:
Class IIa
- If known preexisting bicarbonate-responsive acidosis
- If overdose with tricyclic antidepressants
- To alkalinize the urine in drug overdoses
Class IIb
- If intubated and continued long arrest interval
- Upon return of spontaneous circulation after long arrest interval
Class III
- Hypoxic lactic acidosis

f. If patient remains in asystole or other agonal rhythm after successful intubation and initial medications and no reversible causes are identified, consider termination of resuscitative efforts by a physician. Consider interval since arrest.

ACC/AHA Figure 4

From the American Heart Association. *Advanced Cardiac Life Support,* © American Heart Association, 1997.

Bradycardia Algorithm:
(Patient Is Not in Cardiac Arrest)

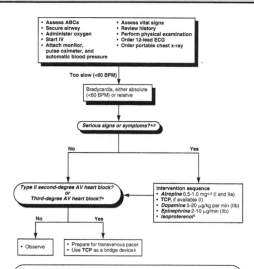

- Assess ABCs
- Secure airway
- Administer oxygen
- Start IV
- Attach monitor, pulse oximeter, and automatic blood pressure

- Assess vital signs
- Review history
- Perform physical examination
- Order 12-lead ECG
- Order portable chest x-ray

Too slow (<60 BPM)

Bradycardia, either absolute (<60 BPM) or relative

Serious signs or symptoms?ᵃ,ᵇ

No — Yes

Type II second-degree AV heart block?
or
Third-degree AV heart block?ᵉ

Intervention sequence
- *Atropine* 0.5-1.0 mgᶜ·ᵈ (I and IIa)
- TCP, if available (I)
- *Dopamine* 5-20 µg/kg per min (IIb)
- *Epinephrine* 2-10 µg/min (IIb)
- *Isoproterenol*ᶠ

No — Yes

- Observe

- Prepare for transvenous pacer
- Use TCP as a bridge deviceᵍ

a. Serious signs or symptoms must be related to the slow rate. Clinical manifestations include
  - Symptoms (chest pain, shortness of breath, decreased level of consciousness)
  - Signs (low BP, shock, pulmonary congestion, CHF, acute MI)

b. Do not delay TCP while awaiting IV access or for *atropine* to take effect if patient is symptomatic.

c. Denervated transplanted hearts will not respond to *atropine*. Go at once to pacing, *catecholamine* infusion, or both.

d. *Atropine* should be given in repeat doses every 3-5 min up to total of 0.03-0.04 mg/kg. Use the shorter dosing interval (3 min) in severe clinical conditions. It has been suggested that *atropine* should be used with caution in atrioventricular (AV) block at the His-Purkinje level (type II AV block and new third-degree block with wide QRS complexes) (Class IIb).

e. Never treat third-degree heart block plus ventricular escape beats with *lidocaine*.

f. *Isoproterenol* should be used, if at all, with extreme caution. At low doses it is Class IIb (possibly helpful); at higher doses it is Class III (harmful).

g. Verify patient tolerance and mechanical capture. Use analgesia and sedation as needed.

ACC/AHA Figure 5
From the American Heart Association. *Advanced Cardiac Life Support,* © American Heart Association, 1997.

Tachycardia Algorithm

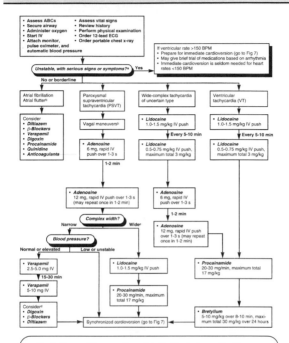

a. Unstable condition must be related to the tachycardia. Signs and symptoms may include chest pain, shortness of breath, decreased level of consciousness, low blood pressure (BP), shock, pulmonary congestion, congestive heart failure, acute myocardial infarction.

b. Carotid sinus pressure is contraindicated in patients with carotid bruits; avoid ice water immersion in patients with ischemic heart disease.

c. If the wide-complex tachycardia is known with certainty to be PSVT and BP is normal/elevated, sequence can include *verapamil*.

d. Use extreme caution with β-blockers after *verapamil*.

ACC/AHA Figure 6
From the American Heart Association. *Advanced Cardiac Life Support*, © American Heart Association, 1997.

Electrical Cardioversion Algorithm: (Patient Is Not in Cardiac Arrest)

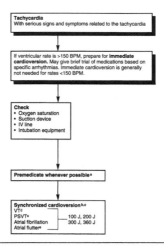

Tachycardia
With serious signs and symptoms related to the tachycardia

If ventricular rate is >150 BPM, prepare for **immediate cardioversion.** May give brief trial of medications based on specific arrhythmias. Immediate cardioversion is generally not needed for rates <150 BPM.

Check
- Oxygen saturation
- Suction device
- IV line
- Intubation equipment

Premedicate whenever possible[a]

Synchronized cardioversion[b,c]
VT[d]
PSVT[e] ————— 100 J, 200 J
Atrial fibrillation   300 J, 360 J
Atrial flutter[e]

---

a. Effective regimens have included a sedative *(eg, **diazepam, midazolam, barbiturates, etomidate, ketamine, methohexital**)* with or without an analgesic agent *(eg, **fentanyl, morphine, meperidine**)*. Many experts recommend anesthesia if service is readily available.

b. Note possible need to resynchronize after each cardioversion.

c. If delays in synchronization occur and clinical conditions are critical, go to immediate unsynchronized shocks.

d. Treat polymorphic VT (irregular form and rate) like VF: 200 J, 200-300 J, 360 J.

e. PSVT and atrial flutter often respond to lower energy levels (start with 50 J).

ACC/AHA Figure 7
From the American Heart Association. *Advanced Cardiac Life Support,* © American Heart Association, 1997.

Acute Pulmonary Edema/Hypotension/ Shock Algorithm

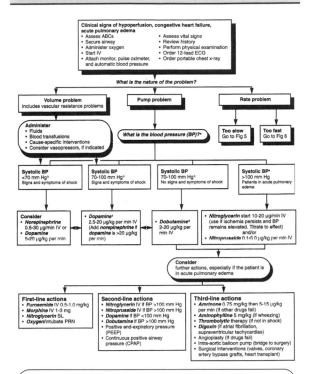

a. Base management after this point on invasive hemodynamic monitoring if possible. Guidelines presume clinical signs of hypoperfusion.

b. Fluid bolus of 250-500 mL normal saline should be tried. If no response, consider sympathomimetics.

c. Move to *dopamine* and stop *norepinephrine* when BP improves. Avoid *dopamine* (consider *dobutamine*) if no signs of hypoperfusion.

d. Add *dopamine* (and avoid *dobutamine*) if systolic BP drops below 90 mm Hg.

e. Consider *nitroglycerin* if initial blood pressures are in this range; reduces preload in patients with acute pulmonary edema.

Acute Myocardial Infarction Algorithm: Recommendations for Early Management of Patients With Chest Pain and Possible Acute Myocardial Infarction

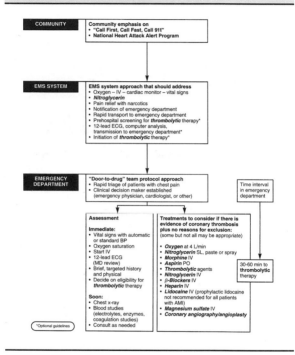

COMMUNITY

Community emphasis on
- "Call First, Call Fast, Call 911"
- National Heart Attack Alert Program

EMS SYSTEM

EMS system approach that should address
- Oxygen – IV – cardiac monitor – vital signs
- *Nitroglycerin*
- Pain relief with narcotics
- Notification of emergency department
- Rapid transport to emergency department
- Prehospital screening for *thrombolytic* therapy*
- 12-lead ECG, computer analysis, transmission to emergency department*
- Initiation of *thrombolytic* therapy*

EMERGENCY DEPARTMENT

"Door-to-drug" team protocol approach
- Rapid triage of patients with chest pain
- Clinical decision maker established (emergency physician, cardiologist, or other)

Time interval in emergency department

Assessment

Immediate:
- Vital signs with automatic or standard BP
- Oxygen saturation
- Start IV
- 12-lead ECG (MD review)
- Brief, targeted history and physical
- Decide on eligibility for *thrombolytic* therapy

Soon:
- Chest x-ray
- Blood studies (electrolytes, enzymes, coagulation studies)
- Consult as needed

*Optional guidelines

Treatments to consider if there is evidence of coronary thrombosis plus no reasons for exclusion: (some but not all may be appropriate)
- *Oxygen* at 4 L/min
- *Nitroglycerin* SL, paste or spray
- *Morphine* IV
- *Aspirin* PO
- *Thrombolytic* agents
- *Nitroglycerin* IV
- *β-Blockers* IV
- *Heparin* IV
- *Lidocaine* IV (prophylactic lidocaine not recommended for all patients with AMI)
- *Magnesium sulfate* IV
- *Coronary angiography/angioplasty*

30-60 min to **thrombolytic** therapy

ACC/AHA Figure 9
From the American Heart Association. *Advanced Cardiac Life Support,* © American Heart Association, 1997.

Ischemic Chest Pain Algorithm

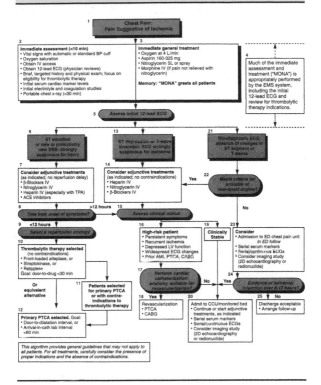

Based on Figures 1,3, 4, and Table 4 in ACC/AHA Guidelines for the management of patients with AMI. J Am Coll Cardiol. 1996;28:1328-1428.

Algorithm for Suspected Stroke Patients

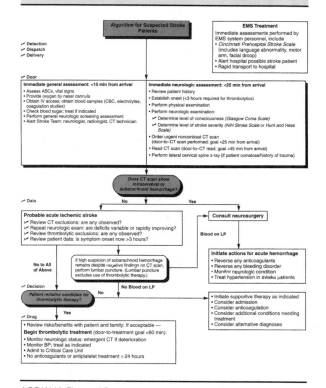

Algorithm for Suspected Stroke Patients

✔ Detection
✔ Dispatch
✔ Delivery

EMS Treatment
Immediate assessments performed by EMS system personnel, include
- *Cincinnati Prehospital Stroke Scale* (includes language abnormality, motor arm, facial droop)
- Alert hospital possible stroke patient
- Rapid transport to hospital

✔ Door

Immediate general assessment: <10 min from arrival
- Assess ABCs, vital signs
- Provide oxygen by nasal cannula
- Obtain IV access; obtain blood samples (CBC, electrolytes, coagulation studies)
- Check blood sugar; treat if indicated
- Perform general neurologic screening assessment
- Alert Stroke Team: neurologist, radiologist, CT technician

Immediate neurologic assessment: <25 min from arrival
- Review patient history
- Establish onset (<3 hours required for thrombolytics)
- Perform physical examination
- Perform neurologic examination:
  ✔ Determine level of consciousness *(Glasgow Coma Scale)*
  ✔ Determine level of stroke severity *(NIH Stroke Scale or Hunt and Hess Scale)*
- Order urgent noncontrast CT scan (door-to-CT scan performed: goal <25 min from arrival)
- Read CT scan (door-to-CT read: goal <45 min from arrival)
- Perform lateral cervical spine x-ray (if patient comatose/history of trauma)

Does CT scan show intracerebral or subarachnoid hemorrhage?

✔ Data   No   Yes

Probable acute ischemic stroke
✔ Review CT exclusions: are any observed?
✔ Repeat neurologic exam: are deficits variable or rapidly improving?
✔ Review thrombolytic exclusions: are any observed?
✔ Review patient data: is symptom onset now >3 hours?

Consult neurosurgery

Blood on LP

No to All of Above

If high suspicion of subarachnoid hemorrhage remains despite negative findings on CT scan, perform lumbar puncture. (Lumbar puncture excludes use of thrombolytic therapy.)

Initiate actions for acute hemorrhage
- Reverse any anticoagulants
- Reverse any bleeding disorder
- Monitor neurologic condition
- Treat hypertension in awake patients

✔ Decision
Patient remains candidate for thrombolytic therapy?   No   No Blood on LP

- Initiate supportive therapy as indicated
- Consider admission
- Consider anticoagulation
- Consider additional conditions needing treatment
- Consider alternative diagnoses

✔ Drug   Yes
- Review risks/benefits with patient and family: If acceptable —
Begin thrombolytic treatment (door-to-treatment goal <60 min):
- Monitor neurologic status: emergent CT if deterioration
- Monitor BP; treat as indicated
- Admit to Critical Care Unit
- No anticoagulants or antiplatelet treatment × 24 hours

ACC/AHA Figure 12
From the American Heart Association. *Advanced Cardiac Life Support,* © American Heart Association, 1997.

Hypothermia Algorithm

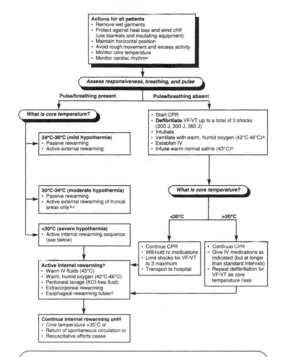

Actions for all patients
- Remove wet garments
- Protect against heat loss and wind chill (use blankets and insulating equipment)
- Maintain horizontal position
- Avoid rough movement and excess activity
- Monitor core temperature
- Monitor cardiac rhythm[a]

Assess responsiveness, breathing, and pulse

Pulse/breathing present

What is core temperature?

34°C-36°C (mild hypothermia)
- Passive rewarming
- Active external rewarming

30°C-34°C (moderate hypothermia)
- Passive rewarming
- Active external rewarming of truncal areas only [b,c]

<30°C (severe hypothermia)
- Active internal rewarming sequence (see below)

Active internal rewarming[b]
- Warm IV fluids (43°C)
- Warm, humid oxygen (42°C-46°C)
- Peritoneal lavage (KCl-free fluid)
- Extracorporeal rewarming
- Esophageal rewarming tubes[d]

Continue internal rewarming until
- Core temperature >35°C or
- Return of spontaneous circulation or
- Resuscitative efforts cease

Pulse/breathing absent
- Start CPR
- **Defibrillate** VF/VT up to a total of 3 shocks (200 J, 300 J, 360 J)
- Intubate
- Ventilate with warm, humid oxygen (42°C-46°C)[b]
- Establish IV
- Infuse warm normal saline (43°C)[b]

What is core temperature?

<30°C
- Continue CPR
- Withhold IV medications
- Limit shocks for VF/VT to 3 maximum
- Transport to hospital

>30°C
- Continue CPR
- Give IV medications as indicated (but at longer than standard intervals)
- Repeat defibrillation for VF/VT as core temperature rises

a. This may require needle electrodes through the skin.

b. Many experts think these interventions should be done only in-hospital, though practice varies.

c. Methods include electric or charcoal warming devices, hot water bottles, heating pads, radiant heat sources, and warming beds.

d. Esophageal rewarming tubes are widely used internationally and should become available in the United States.

ACC/AHA Figure 10
From the American Heart Association. *Advanced Cardiac Life Support,* © American Heart Association, 1997.

6

Heart Failure

Precipitating Factors and Disease States Leading to Heart Failure

PRECIPITATING FACTOR	DISEASE STATE
Infection	Systemic viral or bacterial infection Pericarditis
Endocrine imbalance	Hyperthyroidism Thyroid toxicosis Pheochromocytoma
Nutritional disorder	Beriberi (thiamine disorder) Kwashiorkor (protein deficiency)
Pregnancy	Preeclampsia
Alcoholism	Alcoholic cardiomyopathy
Musculoskeletal disorder	Myasthenia gravis Muscular dystrophy Myotonic dystrophy
Autoimmune disorder	Amyloidosis Sarcoidosis Lupus
Heredity (nonsex-linked autosomal dominant trait)	Hypertrophic cardiomyopathy
Myocardial muscle damage	Coronary artery disease Myocardial infarction
Hemodynamic pressure changes	Hypertension Valve disease (regurgitation or stenosis) Dysrhythmias

Signs and Symptoms of Right-Sided and Left-Sided Heart Failure

RIGHT-SIDED FAILURE	LEFT-SIDED FAILURE
Elevated central venous pressure and right atrial pressure	Elevated pulmonary artery occlusive pressure and left atrial pressure
Jugular venous distention	Dyspnea, paroxysmal nocturnal dyspnea, dyspnea on exertion
Hepatojugular reflex	Orthopnea
Splenomegaly	Adventitious lung sounds: crackles, wheezes, rhonchi
Ascites	Cough, hemoptysis
Nausea and vomiting	Cyanosis
Abdominal distention and anorexia	Cheyne-Stokes breathing
Peripheral edema	Palpitations, cardiac dysrhythmias, tachycardia
Weight gain	Pulsus alternans
Nocturia	Extra heart sounds: S_3, S_4
	Diaphoresis, nocturia

New York Heart Association Functional Classification of Heart Failure

FUNCTIONAL CLASS	DEFINITION	MANIFESTATION
I	Persons with cardiac disease, but without resulting limitations of physical activity	Ordinary physical activity causing no undue fatigue, palpitations, dyspnea, or angina
II	Persons with cardiac disease resulting in slight limitation of physical activity, but comfortable at rest	Ordinary physical activity results in fatigue, palpitations, dyspnea, or angina
III	Persons with cardiac disease resulting in marked limitation of physical activity, but comfortable at rest	Less than ordinary physical activity causes fatigue, palpitations, dyspnea, or angina
IV	Persons with cardiac disease resulting in an inability to carry out any physical activity without discomfort	Symptoms of cardiac insufficiency or of angina often present even at rest

From: The Criteria Committee of the New York Heart Association: (1979). Nomenclature and Criteria for Diagnosis of Diseases of the Heart and Great Vessels. New York, Little, Brown and Company.

Recommended Tests for Patients With Signs or Symptoms of Heart Failure

TEST RECOMMENDATION	FINDING	SUSPECTED DIAGNOSIS
Electrocardiogram	Acute ST–T wave changes	Myocardial ischemia, infarction
	Atrial fibrillation, other tachydysrhythmias	Thyroid disease or heart failure due to rapid ventricular rate
	Bradyarrhythmias	Heart failure due to low heart rate
	Previous MI (e.g., Q waves)	Heart failure due to reduced left ventricular performance
	Low voltage	Pericardial effusion
	Left ventricular hypertrophy	Diastolic dysfunction
Complete blood count	Anemia	Heart failure due to or aggravated by decreased oxygen-carrying capacity

Urinalysis	Proteinuria	Nephrotic syndrome
	Red blood cells or cellular casts	Glomerulonephritis
Serum creatinine	Elevated	Volume overload due to renal failure
Serum albumin	Decreased	Increased extravascular volume due to hypoalbuminemia
T_4 and TSH (obtain only if atrial fibrillation, evidence of thyroid disease, or patient age > 65 years)	Abnormal T_4 or TSH	Heart failure due to or aggravated by hypothyroidism or hyperthyroidism

MI, myocardial infarction; T_4, thyroxine; TSH, thyroid-stimulating hormone.

From Konstam M, Dracup, Baker D, et al: Heart Failure: Evaluation and Care of Patients With Left-Ventricular Systolic Dysfunction, Clinical Practice Guideline No 11. AHCPR Publication No. 94-0612. Rockville, MD: Agency for Health Care Policy and Research, Public Health Service, U.S. Department of Health and Human Services.

Nursing Interventions for Adverse Reactions to Angiotensin-Converting Enzyme (ACE) Inhibitors

ADVERSE REACTIONS	NURSING INTERVENTIONS
Hypotension	Monitor the patient's blood pressure on a regular basis. Blood pressure monitoring is required with the addition of an ACE inhibitor to a regimen that includes diuretics. Instruct the patient that taking the drug at night may reduce the effect of hypotension. Dizziness, fatigue, or lightheadedness should be reported to the patient's practitioner
Hyperkalemia	Potassium levels should be monitored during the initiation of therapy and continued on a regular basis after discharge. Evaluate the relationship between drug therapy and fluid and electrolyte balance. Desired potassium level is 4 0–5.5 mg/ml. Potassium levels >5.5 mg/ml need to be reported to the practitioner
Persistent cough	Evaluate the patient's airway for signs of angioedema and obstruction for which the practitioner needs to be notified. Some coughing is to be expected. Anticipate a dose adjustment when coughing is present
Skin rash	Report skin rash to practitioner. Anticipate a dose adjustment
Renal insufficiency	Monitor creatinine levels in light of electrolyte balance. Creatinine levels greater than 0.5 mg/dl need to be reported

Summary of Medications Commonly Used in Heart Failure

DRUG CLASSIFICATION	GENERIC (TRADE) NAME	INITIAL DOSE (mg)	TARGET DOSE (mg)*	RECOMMENDED MAXIMUM DOSE (mg)
DIURETICS				
Loop	Furosemide (Lasix)	20–40 QD	*	240 BID
Thiazide	Hydrochlorothiazide (Esidrix)	25 QD	*	50 QD
Potassium sparing	Spironolactone (Aldactone)	25 QD	*	100 BID
Carbonic anhydrase inhibitors	Acetazolamide (Diamox)	250–375 QD	*	*
ANGIOTENSION-CONVERTING ENZYME INHIBITORS				
	Captopril (Capoten)	6.25–12.5 TID	50 TID	100 TID
	Enalapril (Vasotec)	2.5 BID	10 BID	20 BID
VASODILATORS				
Nitrates	Intravenous nitroglycerin (Nitro-Bid)	5 µg/min	Titrated as needed	200–400 µg/min
	Isosorbide dinitrate (Isordil)	10 TID	40 TID	80 TID
Other	Hydralazine (Apresoline)	10–25 TID	75 TID	100 TID

* , As needed.

Digoxin Dosing in Heart Failure

PARAMETER	ORAL	INTRAVENOUS
Onset of action	½–2 hr	5–30 min
Peak effect	2–6 hr	1–4 hr
Plasma half-life	32–48 hr	32–48 hr
24-hr loading dose	*Slow:* 0.5–1 mg once a day for 7 days *Rapid:* 0.75–1.25 mg divided into 2 or more doses administered at 6–8 hr intervals	*Rapid:* 0.4–0.6 mg initially, then 0.1–0.3 mg every 6–8 hr as needed
Daily maintenance dose	0.125–0.5 mg in single or divided doses	0.125–0.5 mg in single or divided doses
Therapeutic plasma levels	0.5–2 ng/ml	0.5–2 ng/ml

McKenry L, Salerno E: Mosby's Pharmacology in Nursing. St Louis, Mosby–Year Book, 1995.

Dose, Effect, and Adverse Reactions of Catecholamines Used in Heart Failure

DRUG	ADMINISTRATION GUIDELINES	DOSE	EFFECT	ADVERSE REACTION
Dopamine hydrochloride (Intropin)	*Acute failure:* 1–5 µg/kg/min *Chronic refractory failure:* 0.5–2 µg/kg/min	*Low:* 0.5–2 µg/kg/min	*Low* doses result in primary stimulation of dopaminergic receptors in the renal and mesenteric arteries. Vasodilation promotes increased urinary output	Angina, chest pain, respiratory distress, tachycardia, palpitations, increased heart rate and blood pressure, premature ventricular contractions As the dose increases, so does the likelihood of peripheral vasoconstriction, resulting in pain, mottling, and coldness of extremities
		Moderate: 2–10 µg/kg/min	*Moderate* doses result in primary stimulation of beta₁ adrenergic receptors in the heart, resulting in a positive inotropic effect leading to improved cardiac output	Extravasation of peripheral IV requires administration of phentolamine mesylate (Regitine) to prevent tissue necrosis

(continued)

Dose, Effect, and Adverse Reactions of Catecholamines Used in Heart Failure (continued)

DRUG	ADMINISTRATION GUIDELINES	DOSE	EFFECT	ADVERSE REACTION
Dobutamine hydrochloride (Dobutrex)	2.5–10 μg/kg/min	*High:* >10 μg/kg/min	*High* doses result in primary stimulation of alpha$_1$ adrenergic receptors, promoting increased peripheral resistance and improved blood pressure	Angina or chest pain, respiratory difficulties, and increased heart rate and blood pressure
		2.5–10 μg/kg/min	Primary effect is on beta$_1$ adrenergic fibers, promoting a positive inotropic effect, improving cardiac output	

General Guidelines for Exercise Training of Patients With Heart Failure

Step I: Screen patient for such relative contraindications as

- Symptomatic ventricular tachycardia (VT)
- Active myocarditis
- Pseudoaneurysm

Step II: Exercise testing to set training range and evaluate safety of exercise. Training may be contraindicated in patients with

- Exertional hypotension
- Severe ischemia at low levels of exercise (if possible, revascularization before exercise)
- Sustained exercise-induced VT

Step III: Begin patient's choice of low-level exercise as tolerated 3–4 times a week

- Walking
- Exercise bike
- Low-level weightlifting with 15 repetitions

Step IV: Accelerate program as tolerated with goal set at 45 min at 75% VO_2; more strenuous forms of exercise such as jogging and water aerobics can be added as tolerance improves

Note: *It is not uncommon for a patient who has been exercising for approximately 6 weeks to need an increase in diuretic dosage. Care should be taken that this does not discourage the patient from continuing exercise training.*

From Sullivan M, Hawthorne M: Nonpharmacologic interventions in the treatment of heart failure. J Cardiovasc Nurs 10(2):47–57, 1996.

7

Cardiac Infectious Diseases

Mason's Categories of Myocarditis and Related Organisms

Laboratory Tests in Cardiac Infectious Disease

Summary of Causes of Acute Pericarditis

Comparison of Pain in Pericarditis, Angina, and Myocardial Infarction

Common Organisms in Infective Endocarditis

Common Heart Murmurs Found in Infectious Endocarditis

Mason's Categories of Myocarditis and Related Organisms

CATEGORY	EXAMPLE

ACUTE VIRAL INFECTION

Common	Coxsackievirus A, B1 to B5
	Echovirus
	Human immunodeficiency virus
	Influenza
Less common	Adenovirus
	Epstein-Barr
	Rubeola
	Respiratory syncytial virus
	Rubella
	Varicella-zoster

OTHER INFECTIOUS CAUSES

Bacterial	*Corynebacterium diphtheriae*
	Beta hemolytic streptococci
	Neisseria meningitidis
	Mycoplasma pneumoniae
	Mycobacterium tuberculosis
Protozoal	*Trypanosoma cruzi*
	Toxoplasma gondii
Metazoal	Trichinosis
	Echinococcosis
Fungal	Aspergillosis
	Candidiasis
	Histoplasmosis

HYPERSENSITIVITY TO DRUGS

Anti-infective agents	Amphotericin B
	Isoniazid
	Streptomycin
	Sulfonamides
	Tetracycline
Antihypertensive agents	Methyldopa

AUTOIMMUNE DISEASE

	Systemic lupus erythematosis
	Kawasaki syndrome

LYMPHOCYTIC MYOCARDITIS (POSTVIRAL)

GIANT CELL MYOCARDITIS

Laboratory Tests in Cardiac Infectious Disease

TESTS	PERICARDITIS	ENDOCARDITIS	MYOCARDITIS
White blood cell count	Normal or elevated	Normal or elevated	Elevated
Erythrocyte sedimentation rate	Elevated	Elevated	Elevated
Antibody titers	Antistreptolysin O titers indicated to detect rheumatic fever	Positive antistreptolysin O titer in evidence 6 weeks after onset of disease Hypergammaglobulinemia, circulating immune complexes, low level of serum complement	Antistreptolysin O titers indicated to detect rheumatic fever

Cardiac enzymes, CK/MB fraction	Slightly elevated, especially if in association with myocarditis	Normal	Elevated
Blood urea nitrogen	May be elevated in uremic pericarditis	Normal	Normal
Tuberculosis test	May be positive if tuberculosis pericarditis	Normal	Normal
Cultures	Indicated for pericardial fluid, chest tube drainage	Three or more blood cultures in 24–48 hr identify causative organisms in 90% of patients; negative cultures suggest fungal infection	Stool, throat, pharyngeal washes, and blood to identify bacterial or viral causative organism

Summary of Causes of Acute Pericarditis

CLASSIFICATION	ETIOLOGY	ORGANISM	DISEASE COURSE	POPULATION
Infectious *Idiopathic or viral*	Peak in fall and spring; viral symptoms: fever, chills, fatigue	Coxsackievirus group B, echovirus type B in AIDS patients, CMV, or herpes	Self limiting 1–3 week course, associated with pain; serious complications include acute myocarditis and cardiac tamponade	Opportunistic infection in immunosuppressed patients, e.g., with cancer, AIDS
Bacterial	Associated with mediastinitis after cardiac surgery	*Staphylococcus epidermidis, Staphylococcus* septicemia	Occurs within 1 week of surgery; chest tubes for drainage of purulent material possibly required	Patients experiencing chest trauma or cardiac surgical procedures involving the mediastinum
Postcardiac injury syndrome *Pericarditis after MI (Dressler's syndrome)*	Mediated by an immune response post MI; occurs in less than 5% of MI up to 25% of MI; common findings: fever, fatigue, pericarditis, leukocytosis		2–11 weeks after MI, as early as 1 week, late occurrences up to 1 year, can become chronic	After MI

Postpericardiotomy syndrome	Mediated by immune response; 10%–40% of postcardiac surgery	Occurring within 1 week of surgery or trauma	Cardiac surgical patients and patients who experience trauma of pericardium
Neoplastic	Most common cause of hemorrhagic pericardial effusion; occurs as a result of direct extension of mediastinal tumor, e.g., breast, or through seeding as in leukemia, lymphoma, or melanoma	Varies depending on the length of time the tumor has been growing	Tumor of mediastinum, breast cancer, leukemia, lymphoma, melanoma
Uremic	Seen in renal dialysis patients related to azotemia, develops when blood urea nitrogen > 100 mg/dL; small effusions may be a result of volume overload	Occurs between dialysis; can last 1–2 weeks with large pleural effusions	Patients on renal dialysis

CMV, cytomegalovirus; MI, myocardial infarction.

Comparison of Pain in Pericarditis, Angina, and Myocardial Infarction

CAUSE	LOCATION	CHARACTERISTIC SYMPTOMS	DURATION
Pericarditis	Retrosternal, radiating to arms, neck, back	Stabbing or burning, increasing with inspiration; aggravated by coughing, deep breathing, or lying down; auscultation of a pericardial friction rub	Intermittent
Angina	Substernal, radiating to arms, shoulders, neck, back, or jaw	Burning, squeezing pressure that is mild to severe; onset related to activity, emotional upset, eating a large meal	Short duration, <30 min, relieved by nitroglycerin
Myocardial infarction	Substernal, radiating to arms, shoulder, neck, back, or jaw, particularly on the left side	Heavy pressure, burning, associated with dyspnea, sweating; onset can be related to above, also can be sudden	Prolonged, >30 min, unrelieved by nitroglycerin

Common Organisms in Infective Endocarditis

ORGANISM	ASSOCIATED RISK
GRAM-POSITIVE BACTERIA	
Streptococci	
Alpha hemolytic streptococci	Native valve endocarditis, prosthetic valve endocarditis
Streptococcus bovis	Gastrointestinal malignancies
Enterococci	
Streptococcus faecalis	
Streptococcus durans	
Staphylococci	
Staphylococcus aureus	IV drug abuse
Staphylococcus epidermidis	IV drug abuse
GRAM-NEGATIVE BACTERIA	
Pseudomonas aeruginosa, Serratia murcescens	IV drug abuse, immunocompromised patients, nosocomial infection
HACEK *(Haemophilus* sp., *Actinobacillus actinomycetemcomitans, Cardiobacterium hominis, Eikenella corrodens, Kingella kingae)*	Usually culture negative
FUNGI	
Candida albicans, Candida parapsilosis	IV drug, prosthetic valve endocarditis, cardiac surgery, IV catheters, immunosuppression

Common Heart Murmurs Found in Infectious Endocarditis

TYPE	TIMING	LOCATION	CONFIGURATION	INTENSITY	PITCH	QUALITY	RADIATION
Aortic stenosis	Systole; sound begins shortly after S_1, ends before S_2	Second right intercostal space (loudest); Erb's point (third left intercostal space along the sternal border); apex	Crescendo/ decrescendo	Sometimes soft, often loud, with a thrill, heard best with patient sitting and leaning forward	Medium at apex	Harsh, may be more musical at apex	Carotid arteries, usually the right; down left sternal border, even to apex
Aortic regurgitation	Early diastole; immediately after S_1	Second to fourth left intercostal space	Decrescendo	Grades I–III, best heard with patient sitting, leaning forward with breath held in exhalation	High	Blowing	Lower left sternal border

Mitral regurgitation	Systole, begins with S_1 and continues to S_2	Apex	Holosystolic	Soft to loud; does not become louder on inspiration	Medium to high	Blowing	Left axilla, less often to left sternal border
Mitral valve prolapse	Mid to late systole, clicks are heard in midsystole (position changes will affect timing)	Apex, often lateralized	Crescendo	Varies with position changes; squatting may intensify	High	Whooping, honking	Varies
Mitral stenosis	Diastole, between S_1 and S_2	Apex	Decrescendo/crescendo	Grades I-IV; louder in left lateral supine position or after exercise; heard better in exhalation	Low	Rumbling	Little or none

From Matthews D: The prevention and diagnosis of infective endocarditis. Nurse Pract 19:55, 1994. © Springhouse Corporation, Springhouse, PA.

8

Cardiac Surgery and Heart Transplantation

Preoperative Educational Content for Cardiac Surgery

EXPECTATIONS BEFORE CARDIAC SURGERY

Diagnostic tests (chest x-ray, laboratory studies)
Skin preparation
NPO at least 8 hr preoperatively
Ability to demonstrate effective cough and deep
    breathing, using splint for sternal or chest support
Ability to demonstrate use of incentive spirometry
Ability to demonstrate leg exercises (foot flexion and
    extension)
Time family members should be at the hospital to
    visit preoperatively

EXPECTATIONS DURING CARDIAC SURGERY

Type of procedure that is anticipated
Anticipated time in the operating room
Convenient location for family to wait during surgery
How family will be contacted at intervals during surgery
    and/or after surgery is completed

EXPECTATIONS AFTER CARDIAC SURGERY

Name and location of ICU
External devices to expect and their purpose
    Endotracheal tube and ventilator
    Nasogastric tube
    ECG electrodes and monitoring
    Hemodynamic monitoring (pulmonary artery and
        arterial lines)
    Epicardial pacing wires and external pulse generator
    Chest tubes and drainage system
    Foley catheter
Procedures to expect
    Endotracheal suctioning if intubated
    Pain management plan
    Blood administration
    Activity progression

ADDITIONAL EXPECTATIONS

Sounds of ICU
Family involvement

Cardiopulmonary Bypass System

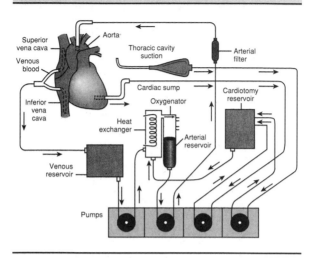

Pharmacologic Agents Used to Control Postoperative Bleeding

MEDICATION	ACTION	DOSAGE
Desmopressin (DDAVP)	Increases release of factor VIII and improves platelet function	0.3–0.4 µg/kg in 50 mL normal saline over 15–30 min
Aprotinin (Trasylol)	Antifibrinolytic; stabilizes fibrin clots, preserves platelet function	15–20,000 KIU/ kg loading; 50,000 KIU/hr infusion
Aminocaproic acid	Antifibrinolytic; stabilizes fibrin clots	5 g loading over 1 hr; 1–1.25 g/hr infusion (maximum dose 30 g in 24 hr)
Tranexamic acid	Antifibrinolytic; stabilizes fibrin clot	10–15 mg/kg or 0.5–1 g IV every 4–6 hr

Adapted from Auer IK: The role of pharmacologic agents in blood conservation. AACN Clin Iss 7:262, 1996.

Educational Content for Patients Preparing for Home After Cardiac Surgery

Pain management

Incision care

Rest and activity program, including initiation of a cardiac rehabilitation program, if appropriate

Low-fat, low-cholesterol diet (sodium restrictions may or may not apply)

Medications

Signs and symptoms to report to physician (e.g., increase in weight, chest pain, dyspnea, nocturnal dyspnea, cough, edema)

Risk factor modification

Standard Evaluation Testing Determination of Heart Transplantation Candidacy

EVALUATION TESTS	INDICATIONS
Metabolic VO_2 stress test	Evaluate heart failure class to predict survival
Echocardiogram/ multigated angiogram	Evaluate heart function, degree of regurgitation, and left ventricular ejection fraction
Left heart catheterization	R/O reversible coronary artery disease
Right heart catheterization	R/O nonreversible elevated pulmonary vascular resistance
Pulmonary function test	R/O obstructive disease, primary lung disorder
Vascular studies (peripheral and carotid)	R/O arterial stenosis in lower extremities or carotids
Ultrasound (abdomen and retroperitoneum)	R/O masses, abdominal aortic aneurysms, and gallstones; evaluate kidney size
Posteroanterior and lateral chest radiographs	R/O masses or effusions
Mammogram (females)	R/O masses
Dental medicine consult	R/O infection

(continued)

Standard Evaluation Testing Determination of Heart Transplantation Candidacy (continued)

EVALUATION TESTS	INDICATIONS
Psychosocial consult	R/O unstable psychiatric history; evaluate compliance, transportation, and support systems
Finance consult	R/O need for financial assistance, fund raising
Physical therapy consult	R/O disabling factors; evaluate rehabilitation needs
Dietary consult	R/O morbid obesity or cachexia
Purified protein derivative test	R/O tuberculosis exposure
Gynecologic examination	R/O cancer
LABORATORY TESTING	
HIV, hepatitis screen	R/O active or chronic infection
Type and screen	R/O donor incompatibility
Cytomegalovirus, herpes simplex virus, varicella-zoster virus, Epstein-Barr virus, *Toxoplasma* titers	R/O active infections, susceptibility to infection after transplant
Prostate surface antigen (males)	R/O prostate cancer (screening)
Tissue typing	R/O need for prospective crossmatch
Urinalysis/urine culture	R/O infection
24-hr urine collection	R/O renal insufficiency

Contraindications to Listing Heart Transplantation Patients

Absolute Contraindications

- Malignancy
- Positive HIV test
- Sepsis
- End-organ disease due to uncontrolled diabetes

Relative Contraindications

- Age
- Pulmonary infarction in the past 8 weeks
- Diabetes
- Vascular disease

- Major chronic disabling illness (e.g., lupus or stroke with residual deficits)
- Active mental illness
- Fixed pulmonary vascular resistance >600
- Nonreversible vital organ impairment (e.g., primary pulmonary, liver, or kidney disease not due to low-output state)

- Obesity
- Drug, tobacco, or alcohol use
- Peptic ulcer disease

United Network of Organ Sharing (UNOS) Current and Proposed Criteria for Listing Patients

STATUS		CRITERIA
CURRENT		
1	Must meet one criterion	IV inotropes and in an intensive care unit
		Mechanical support (IABP, ventricular assist device, or ventilator) and in the ICU
		Thermo Cardiosystems Internal left ventricular assist device in the hospital or at home
2	Must meet one criterion	IV inotropes but not in the ICU (including home-bound patients)
		Intensive care bound but not on IV inotropes or mechanical support
		Maintained on oral medications at home or in the hospital
PROPOSED		
1a	Must meet *all* three criteria	Admitted in the listing transplant center or hospital
		Hemodynamic monitoring
		Cardiac support (IV inotropes, IABP, ventricular assist device)

(continued)

United Network of Organ Sharing (UNOS) Current and Proposed Criteria for Listing Patients (continued)

STATUS		CRITERIA
1b	Must meet one criterion	Circulatory assist device (these patients can be at home)
		ICU with IV inotropes
2a	Must meet *one* criterion	IV inotropes not in an ICU (can be at home)
		Intensive care, no support
2b		All other patients listed, typically patients at home on oral medications

IABP, intraaortic balloon pump.

From The United Network for Organ Sharing: Policy and By-Law Proposals. Richmond, VA, UNOS, 1100 Boulders Parkway, Suite 500, PO Box 13770, Richmond, VA 23225-8770, August 1, 1997.

Donor Information Used to Determine Acceptable Candidates

- Brain death criteria met with corresponding consent for donation
- Cause of death
- Past medical history: no evidence of cancer
- Social history: no heavy alcohol, smoking, or drug use
- Recent hospital course events: no septicemia
- Hemodynamics: no circulatory arrest or minimal interruption of cardiac output
- Laboratory data: negative for HIV and hepatitis B; recipient patients who are hepatitis C–positive can receive hepatitis C–positive donor hearts
- Blood type
- Donor size (height and weight)
- Electrocardiogram
- Echocardiogram
- Cardiac catheterization (requested if the donor is older than 50 years or has a history of smoking, diabetes, or hypertension)

Long-Term Immunosuppression

IMMUNOSUPPRESSIVE AGENT	PILL STRENGTH	LABORATORY LEVELS
Cyclosporine (Sandimmune or Neoral)	100-mg and 25-mg gel capsules (cannot be broken)	Maintain cyclosporine trough level at: 250–300 mg/L the first year 200–250 mg/L the second year 150–200 mg/L thereafter Monitor for increase in creatinine, liver function tests
Tacrolimus (Prograf)	4-mg, 2-mg, and 1-mg capsules (cannot be broken)	Tacrolimus trough level: 15–20 mg/L
Azathioprine (Imuran)	50-mg tablets (can be broken in half)	WBC 4000–8000 Monitor for drop in WBC, hemoglobin, or platelets *(continued)*

Long-Term Immunosuppression (continued)

IMMUNOSUPPRESSIVE AGENT	PILL STRENGTH	LABORATORY LEVELS
Mycophenylate mofetil (CellCept)	500-mg and 250-mg capsules (cannot be broken)	WBC 4000–8000 Monitor for drop in WBC, hemoglobin, or platelets
Prednisone (Deltasone)	10-mg, 5-mg, 2-mg, and 1-mg pills (can be broken in half)	Per program taper protocol Monitor fasting glucose level for signs of steroid-induced diabetes

WBC, white blood cell count.

Side Effects From Immunosuppressive Therapy for Heart Transplantation Patients

MEDICATION	SIDE EFFECTS
Cyclosporine (Sandimmune, Neoral)	Hypertension Nephrotoxicity Hypercholesterolemia Hepatoxicity Hyperkalemia Hyperglycemia	Tremors Seizures Headache Gingival hyperplasia Hirsutism Nausea Vomiting
FK506 Tacrolimus (Prograf)	Hypertension Nephrotoxicity Hyperkalemia Hyperglycemia Headache	Tremors Seizures Nausea Diarrhea
Prednisone (Deltasone)	Joint pain Muscle weakness Increased appetite Salt and water retention Increased weight Hypertension Hyperglycemia, diabetes Cushingoid appearance (moon face)	Mood swings Insomnia Night sweats Gastrointestinal ulceration Cataracts Hirsutism Acne Ultraviolet ray sensitivity (need SPF >15 sunscreen)

(continued)

Side Effects From Immunosuppressive Therapy for Heart Transplantation Patients (continued)

MEDICATION	SIDE EFFECTS
Azathioprine (Imuran)	Bone marrow suppression (particularly WBC and occasionally RBC) Bruising Alopecia Hepatotoxicity
Mycophenylate mofetil (CellCept)	Abdominal pain Nausea Vomiting Diarrhea Leukopenia Neutropenia Sepsis (typically cytomegalovirus)
OKT3	Rigors Malaise Pyrexia Diarrhea Hypertension Hypotension Pulmonary edema Meningitis
Antilymphocyte preparation (Atgam)	Fever Chills Serum sickness Inflammatory reactions Bone marrow suppression Thrombocytopenia Anaphylaxis

Common Infections After Transplantation

Viral

Cytomegalovirus
Epstein-Barr virus
Herpes simplex virus
Varicella-zoster virus

Bacterial

Nosocomial
Pneumococcal pneumonia
Nocardia

Protozoal and Fungal

Candida
Pneumocystis
Aspergillus
Toxoplasma
Cryptococcus

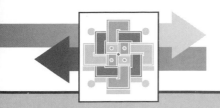

Respiratory System

9

Respiratory Anatomy and Physiology

Anterior (A) and Posterior (B) Anatomic Views

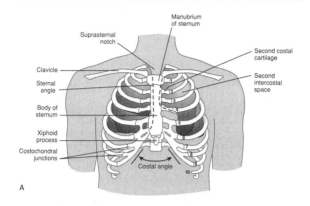

A

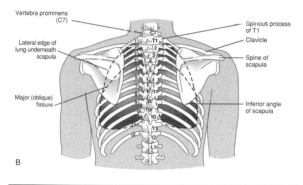

B

Interior Lung View

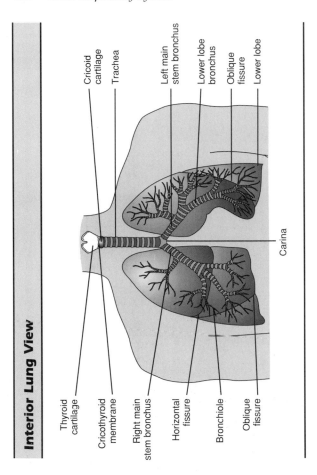

Thyroid cartilage

Cricothyroid membrane

Right main stem bronchus

Horizontal fissure

Bronchiole

Oblique fissure

Cricoid cartilage

Trachea

Left main stem bronchus

Lower lobe bronchus

Oblique fissure

Lower lobe

Carina

Pulmonary Circulation

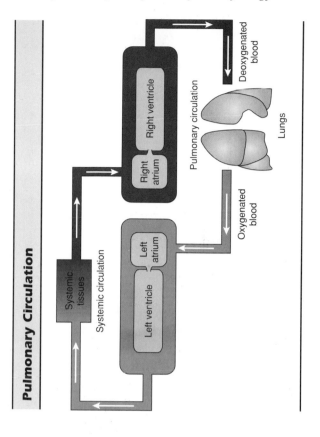

Four Volumes of Ventilatory Function

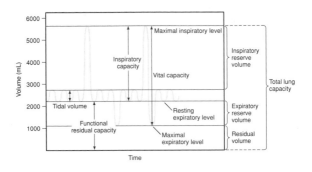

From Hansen M: Pathophysiology. Philadelphia, WB Saunders, Co., 1998.

Diffusion of Oxygen from Alveolus into Pulmonary Capillary

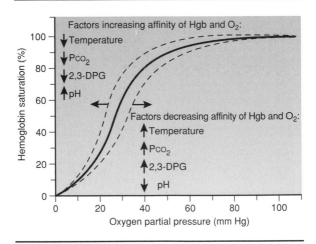

Carbon Dioxide Transportation

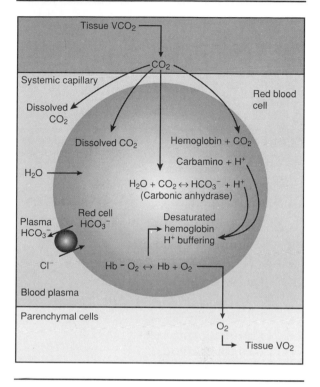

10

Respiratory Assessment

Specific Characteristics to Assess Regarding Cough

Specific Areas of Assessment During Inspiration

Factors Influencing Tactile Fremitus

Description of Types of Chest Pain Related to the Respiratory System

LOCATION	CHARACTERISTICS	POSSIBLE CAUSES
Musculoskeletal	Sharply localized point tenderness worsened by deep breathing, cough, sneezing	Thoracic incision; muscle, ligament strains; rib fracture; lesions on the ribs; tumors
Pleuropulmonary	Sharply localized stabbing in lateral aspect of chest; may be sudden in onset aggravated by movement, cough, deep breathing; may radiate pain to shoulder, abdomen	Pleurisy, pneumothorax
Airways	Sudden onset; crushing midsternal pain, may be pleuritic as well; mimics myocardial pain	Acute pulmonary embolism; depending on the severity of the embolism, chest pain may be located over the affected side or area of the lung
	Burning, soreness midsternal area	Acute tracheobronchitis

Description of Abnormal Breathing Patterns

ABNORMAL BREATHING PATTERN	DESCRIPTION
Tachypnea	A breathing rate faster than 20 breaths per minute. Nonspecific finding that may be due to a variety of causes, including pain, anxiety, fever, hypercapnia, or hypoxemia
Bradypnea	A breathing pattern slower than 10 breaths per minute. Nonspecific finding that may be due to a variety of causes, including excessive sedatives or narcotics, metabolic disorders, or brain disorders
Apnea	Disruption and cessation of air flow to the lungs. Usually considered pathologic if greater than 15 seconds. Prolonged apnea may occur due to respiratory arrest due to acute upper airway obstruction, stroke, or depression of the respiratory center
Cheyne–Stokes	A crescendo/decrescendo pattern of breathing of progressively deeper respirations followed by progressively more shallow respirations. This is followed by a period of apnea. Then the cycle repeats itself. Periods of apnea may last up to 15–20 seconds. Caused by changes in blood flow to the respiratory center or impairment in the control of breathing
Kussmaul	Deep, regular breaths at a rate greater than 20 breaths per minute. Caused by the respiratory system reacting to a severe metabolic acidotic state. The respiratory system attempts to compensate by excreting CO_2 in response to the metabolic acidosis
Biot's	Irregular breathing with an unpredictable rate, pattern, and depth. May include periods of apnea. Due to central nervous system disorder affecting the central control of breathing (head trauma, stroke). This pattern is not compatible with life and will require intubation and mechanical ventilation

Modified from Kersten LD: Comprehensive Respiratory Nursing. Philadelphia, WB Saunders Co., 1989.

Percussion Notes and Their Characteristics

	AMPLITUDE	PITCH	QUALITY	DURATION	SAMPLE LOCATION
Resonant	Medium loud	Low	Clear, hollow	Moderate	Over normal lung tissue
Hyperresonant	Louder	Lower	Booming	Longer	Normal over child's lung; in the adult, over lungs with abnormal amount of air, as in emphysema

	Loud	High	Musical and drumlike (like the kettle drum)	Sustained longest	Over air-filled viscus, e.g., the stomach, the intestine
Tympany					
Dull	Soft	High	Muffled thud	Short	Relatively dense organ, as liver or spleen
Flat	Very soft	High	A dead stop of sound, absolute dullness	Very short	When no air is present, over thigh muscles, bone, or tumor

From Jarvic C: Physical Examination and Health Assessment, 2nd ed. Philadelphia, WB Saunders Co., 1996.

Examples of Patient Situations Leading to False-Positive Lung Sounds

PATIENT SITUATION	FALSE-POSITIVE LUNG SOUND	EXPLANATION	TO ELIMINATE SOUND
Mechanical ventilation	Rhonchi, usually expiratory	Water bubbling in ventilator tubings	Empty ventilator tubings before auscultation
Pursed-lip breathing	Decreased breath sounds (expiration almost absent)	Mouth closed during expiration	Instruct patient to exhale with mouth wide open
Nasogastric tube	High- or low-pitched squeak, anterior chest	Varies with intermittent suction	Clamp nasogastric tube during auscultation
Chest hair	Crackles or other extraneous sounds	Hair moves against diaphragm during chest movement	Select areas free of hair or wet chest hair before auscultation
Stethoscope contact with patient's gown, bedsheets, etc.	Crackles or other extraneous sounds	Articles rub against stethoscope, diaphragm, or tubing	Do not listen over clothes or allow any part of stethoscope to touch articles of clothing
Muscle tension, as in Shivering Muscle twitching Pain Use of accessory muscles of respiration	Crackles or other extraneous sounds Decreased breath sounds	Increased surface tension Breathing is not free and easy	May be unavoidable Listen after sedation or pain medication Instruct tense patient to relax shoulders

Modified from Kersten LD: Comprehensive Respiratory Nursing. Philadelphia, WB Saunders Co, 1989.

Characteristics of Normal Breath Sounds

SOUND	PITCH	AMPLITUDE	DURATION	QUALITY	NORMAL LOCATION
Bronchial (tracheal)	High	Loud	Inspiration < expiration	Harsh, hollow, tubular	Trachea and larynx
Bronchovesicular	Moderate	Moderate	Inspiration = expiration	Mixed	Over major bronchi where fewer alveoli are located; posterior, between scapulae, especially on right; anterior, around upper sternum in first and second intercostal spaces

(continued)

Characteristics of Normal Breath Sounds (continued)

SOUND	PITCH	AMPLITUDE	DURATION	QUALITY	NORMAL LOCATION
Vesicular	Low	Soft	Inspiration > expiration	Rustling, like the sound of the wind in the trees	Over peripheral lung fields where air flows through smaller bronchioles and alveoli

From Jarvis C: Physical Examination and Health Assessment, 2nd ed. Philadelphia, WB Saunders Co, 1996.

Disorders Causing Decreased or Absent Breath Sounds

DECREASED	ABSENT	DECREASED OR ABSENT
Hypoventilation	Respiratory arrest	Pleural effusion
Pleural thickening	Pneumonectomy	Hemothorax
Obesity	Elevated diaphragm	Pneumothorax
Chest cage deformity	Large abdomen	Empyema
Emphysema	Stomach distention	Malpositioned endotracheal tube
Pulmonary embolism	Paralyzed diaphragm	Partial to complete airway obstruction
Partial airway obstruction	Large lung resection	Tumor
Tumor	Atelectasis	Foreign object
Foreign object	Complete airway obstruction	Pneumonia
Left ventricular failure	Tumor	Upper airway obstruction
Pneumonia	Foreign object	Atelectasis
Atelectasis	Laryngeal spasm	Pulmonary cavitation
	Mucous plugs	
	Collapsed lung	

From Kersten LD: Comprehensive Respiratory Nursing, Philadelphia, WB Saunders Co., 1989.

Characteristics of Abnormal or Adventitious Lung Sounds

SOUND	DESCRIPTION	MECHANISM	CLINICAL EXAMPLE
DISCONTINUOUS SOUNDS			
Crackles—fine (rales) 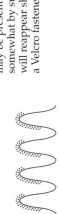 Inspiration Expiration	Discontinuous, high-pitched, short crackling, popping sounds heard during inspiration that are not cleared by coughing; you can simulate this sound by rolling a strand of hair between your fingers near your ear, or by moistening your thumb and index finger and separating them near your ear	Inhaled air collides with previously deflated airways; airways suddenly pop open, creating crackling sound as gas pressures between the two compartments equalize	*Late inspiratory crackles* occur with restrictive disease: pneumonia, congestive heart failure, and interstitial fibrosis *Early inspiratory crackles* occur with obstructive disease: chronic bronchitis, asthma, and emphysema
Crackles—coarse (coarse rales)	Loud, low-pitched bubbling and gurgling sounds that start in early inspiration and may be present in expiration; may decrease somewhat by suctioning or coughing but will reappear shortly; sound like opening a Velcro fastener	Inhaled air collides with secretions in the trachea and large bronchi	Pulmonary edema, pneumonia, pulmonary fibrosis; also heard in the terminally ill who have a depressed cough reflex

156

Atelectatic crackles
(atelectatic rales)

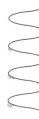

Sound like fine crackles, but do not last and are disappear after the first few breaths; heard in axillae and bases (usually dependent) of lungs

When sections of alveoli are not fully aerated, they deflate and accumulate secretions; crackles are heard when these sections re-expand with a few deep breaths

In aging adults, bed-ridden persons, or persons just aroused from sleep

Pleural friction rub

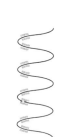

A very superficial sound that is coarse and low pitched; it has a grating quality as if two pieces of leather are being rubbed together; sounds just like crackles, but *close* to the ear; sounds louder if you push the stethoscope harder onto the chest wall; sound is inspiratory and expiratory

Caused when pleurae become inflamed and lose their normal lubricating fluid; their opposing roughened pleural surfaces rub together during respiration; heard best in anterolateral wall where greatest lung mobility exists

Pleuritis, accompanied by pain with breathing (rub disappears after a few days if pleural fluid accumulates and separates pleurae)

(continued)

Characteristics of Abnormal or Adventitious Lung Sounds (continued)

SOUND	DESCRIPTION	MECHANISM	CLINICAL EXAMPLE
CONTINUOUS SOUNDS			
Wheeze—high-pitched (sibilant)	High-pitched, musical squeaking sounds that sound polyphonic (multiple notes as in a musical chord); predominate in expiration but may occur in both expiration and inspiration	Air squeezed or compressed through passageways narrowed almost to closure by collapsing, swelling, secretions, or tumors; the passageway walls oscillate in apposition between the closed and barely open positions; the resulting sound is similar to that of a vibrating reed	Diffuse airway obstruction from acute asthma or chronic emphysema
Wheeze—low-pitched (sonorous rhonchi)	Low-pitched, monophonic (single note), musical snoring, moaning sounds; they are heard throughout the cycle, although they are more prominent on expiration; may clear somewhat by coughing	Airflow obstruction as described by the vibrating reed mechanism above; the pitch of the wheeze cannot be correlated with the size of the passageway that generates it	Bronchitis, single bronchus obstruction from airway tumor

158

Stridor

High-pitched, monophonic, inspiratory, crowing sound; louder in neck than over chest wall

Originating in larynx or trachea; upper airway obstruction from swollen, inflamed tissues or lodged foreign body

Croup and acute epiglottitis in children, post-extubation edema, and foreign inhalation; obstructed airway may be life-threatening

Although nothing in clinical practice seems to differ more than the nomenclature of adventitious sounds, most authorities concur on two categories: (1) discontinuous, discrete crackling sounds and (2) continuous, or musical, sounds.

From Jarvis C: Physical Examination and Health Assessment, 2nd ed. Philadelphia, WB Saunders Co., 1996.

Summary of Physical Assessment Findings in Common Respiratory Diseases

PROBLEM	INSPECTION	PALPATION	PERCUSSION	AUSCULTATION
Chronic obstructive pulmonary disease exacerbation	Increased anteroposterior diameter of chest; if hypoxemic, central cyanosis; most comfortable in sitting position with stabilization of shoulder girdle (tripod position); use of accessory muscles; labored respiration; pursed-lip breathing; prolonged expiration	↓Movement ↓Fremitus with air trapping	Hyperresonant	Distant breath sounds if not moving air well; crackles, rhonchi, or wheezes
Asthma exacerbation	Most comfortable in sitting position with stabilization of shoulder girdle (tripod position); use of accessory muscles; labored respiration; pursed-lip breathing; central cyanosis	↓Movement ↓Fremitus with air trapping	Hyperresonant	Wheezes, distant breath sounds if not moving air well

				Crackles
Atelectasis	Symmetry of chest wall movement unless segment or lobe involved; depending on severity, respiratory rate may be increased	Minor, no change; major, asymmetry of chest wall movement	Dull over affected area	Crackles
Pneumonia	Tachypnea, labored breathing, use of accessory muscles; may have cough, sputum production, fever; depending upon respiratory compromise, may have central cyanosis	Asymmetric chest wall movement; ↑fremitus over affected area	Dull	Bronchial breath sounds over area of consolidation; crackles, rhonchi
Pneumothorax	Tachypnea, labored breathing, possible central cyanosis, use of accessory muscles	↓Movement affected side, ↓fremitus	Hyperresonant	Diminished; absent over area of collapse
Tension pneumothorax	Tachypnea, labored breathing, central cyanosis; use of accessory muscles; tracheal shift	↓Movement affected side, ↓fremitus	Tympany	Diminished; absent over affected area

(continued)

Summary of Physical Assessment Findings in Common Respiratory Diseases (continued)

PROBLEM	INSPECTION	PALPATION	PERCUSSION	AUSCULTATION
Pulmonary edema	Tachypnea, labored breathing, frothy sputum production	Normal or decreased chest wall movement	Normal or dull (depends on severity)	Fine, coarse crackles (initially in dependent areas of lung)
Pleural effusion	Tachypnea, labored breathing	↓Movement affected side, ↓fremitus	Dull	Diminished; absent over area of effusion

Respiratory Historical Assessment

Chief complaint
Medicine allergies
History of present illness: Determine if the critical
    care admission is related to
    Acute vs. chronic respiratory problem
      Duration of problem/disease process
      Previous hospitalization for a similar problem
    Respiratory complication of surgery or of another
      disease process
    Respiratory comorbidity

Past respiratory history
    Chronic obstructive lung disease or chronic
      obstructive pulmonary disease (emphysema,
      chronic bronchitis, bronchiectasis, cystic
      fibrosis)
    Asthma
    Frequent infections—sinusitis, upper respiratory or
      lower respiratory infections
    Pneumonia
    Tuberculosis; when was the patient's most recent
      tuberculosis test

Past surgical history
    Any previous surgeries related to the lung, thorax
    With these surgeries, were there any problems with
      general anesthesia, lung problems after surgery,
      or the need for mechanical ventilation

Medications
    Present medications (prescription, nonprescription
      [over the counter], inhalers, cutaneous patches,
      oxygen, nebulizer treatments, home remedies)
    Indication, dosage, schedule, time since last dose
    Recently discontinued medications
    Recent vaccines (flu, Pneumovax, others)

Allergies
Social history
    Smoking history
      Nonsmoker, active smoker, or exsmoker
      Type of smoking history: cigarettes, cigars, pipe
      Duration of smoking history (years) and packs
        per day
      Pack year history (PYH) = duration in years ×
        average no. of packs per day
      Smoking cessation history
    Ethyl alcohol intake

(continued)

Respiratory Historical Assessment (continued)

Family history of respiratory problems

Symptom assessment
  Breathlessness, shortness of breath
  Cough
  Sputum production
  Hemoptysis
  Chest pain

Assessment of History of Acute or Chronic Respiratory Problems

1. Have you ever been treated by a doctor or health-care provider for a lung problem (outpatient, emergency room, inpatient)?
2. Have you ever been attached to a breathing machine (ventilator) or had a tube placed into your mouth or nose to help you breathe?
3. Have you ever had any breathing test that measures the amount of air in your lungs or a blood test to look at the amount of oxygen in your blood?
4. Do you take any medicines to help your breathing?

Respiratory Symptoms: Specific Characteristics to Assess

Key Pulmonary Symptom	Characteristics to Assess for Each Symptom
Breathlessness (dyspnea, shortness of breath) Cough Sputum production Hemoptysis Chest pain	Location Quality Related symptoms Severity Timing

Specific Assessment Questions to Be Asked Regarding Breathlessness

Location	How does the breathlessness feel? Where is it located?
Quality	Is it an acute or a chronic symptom? Is it intermittent or continuous? Is it increasing, decreasing, or staying the same?
Related symptoms	Are there other signs of respiratory distress or problems? (e.g., pursed-lip breathing, use of accessory muscles, central cyanosis, increased respiratory rate, increased inspiratory/ expiratory ratio, chest pain)
Severity	Are you able to complete a sentence or speak only in short phrases? Are you reluctant to speak due to the breathlessness? What position do you usually assume? Are you able to lie flat in bed? How many pillows do you use at night? Have you ever used supplemental oxygen?
Timing	How long have you experienced shortness of breath? Is it intermittent or continuous? Are you short of breath at rest or with exercise (quantify the amount—number of feet walked, number of stairs, etc.)? Attempt to differentiate between shortness of breath and fatigue as a limiting factor.

Specific Characteristics to Assess Regarding Cough

Location	Location more upper airway (throat clearing) or deeper, lower airway in nature
Quality	Type: dry or "hacking" vs. productive Productivity: amount, color, characteristics of sputum
Related symptoms	Accompanying signs or symptoms (breathlessness, fever, night sweats, weight loss, nausea, vomiting, chest pain, dizziness, wheezing)
Severity	Presence of paroxysms of cough (uncontrollable spasms of cough) Impairment of activities of daily living, quality of life Medications associated with cough or taken to relieve the cough (over the counter, prescribed)
Timing	Duration of the cough; acute onset or chronic problem Frequency, occurrence during the day and night Association with an activity or event (eating, drinking fluids, lying flat) Relationship with any environmental factors Has patient had recent instrumentation of the airway (intubation, bronchoscopy, surgical procedure involving airways)

Specific Areas of Assessment During Inspiration

General	Level of consciousness
	General nutritional status (cachexia, obesity)
	Skin turgor
	Musculoskeletal development
	Positioning of patient
	Speech pattern, ability to speak in sentences
	Hoarseness
	Scars
Extremities	Edema
	Peripheral cyanosis
	Clubbing
Head and neck	Type of breathing (mouth vs. nose)
	Rate, pattern of breathing; inspiratory/expiratory ratio
	Nasal flaring
	Pursed-lip breathing
	Central cyanosis
	Tracheal positioning
	Use of accessory muscles of shoulders and neck
Thorax	Rate and pattern of breathing
	Symmetry of chest wall movement
	Synchrony of chest and abdominal movements
	Chest wall deformities
	Bulging, retraction of interspaces

Factors Influencing Tactile Fremitus

Factors influencing normal intensity of tactile fremitus

Location of bronchi to chest wall
Thickness of chest wall
Conditions that increase density of lung tissue

Increased fremitus

Thin chest wall
Lung consolidation, pneumonia
Severe atelectasis
Lung mass

Decreased fremitus

Obesity
Muscular chest wall
Conditions with air trapping (chronic obstructive
    pulmonary disease, asthma)
Pleural effusion
Pneumothorax
Pleural thickening

Respiratory Laboratory and Diagnostic Tests

169

Acid–Base Definitions

Acid	Ion that releases H^+ in solution
Base	Ion that combines with H^+ and removes it from solution
pH	Symbol used to express the concentration of H^+; pH is the negative logarithm of H^+ ion concentration; an inverse relationship
Acidemia	pH < 7.35
Alkalemia	pH > 7.45
Acidosis	Process leading to state of excess addition of H^+ or a loss of basic ions from a solution, $\downarrow$**pH**
Alkalosis	Process leading to state of excess removal of H^+ or the addition of basic ions to solution, $\uparrow$**pH**
Compensatory mechanisms	Responses of chemical buffers or respiratory or renal system

Characteristics of pH

Normal	7.35–7.45 (arterial)

$$pH = \frac{HCO_3^-\ \text{(bicarbonate, kidney)}}{H_2CO_3\ \text{(carbonic acid,* lung)}}$$

Acidemia	pH < 7.35 (excess H^+)
Alkalemia	pH > 7.45 (deficit H^+)

*Carbonic acid = $P_{CO_2} \times 0.0301$.

Physiologic Effects of Acidemia and Alkalemia

EFFECTS OF ACIDEMIA (pH < 7.35)	EFFECTS OF ALKALEMIA (pH > 7.45)
Cardiopulmonary	
Pulmonary vascular constriction	Bronchoconstriction
Myocardial irritability, decreased contractility	Pulmonary vascular dilation
Systemic vasodilation	Myocardial irritability
	Systemic vasoconstriction
CNS	
Depressed cortical function	Constricted cerebral vessels
Dilated cerebral vessels	Increased excitability of neuromuscular system
Changes in respiratory control center	
Associated Symptoms	
Headache	Dizziness
Slow responses	Tingling of fingers or toes
Asterixis (flapping tremor)	Muscle weakness or spasm
Confusion	Sweating
Nausea, vomiting	Dysrhythmias
Kussmaul's breathing	

Characteristics of $Paco_2$

Normal: 35–45 mm Hg
Respiratory/ventilatory parameter
Regulated by the lung
Think of CO_2 as an acid
Alveolar hypoventilation: $\uparrow CO_2$ (hypercarbia, hypercapnia)
Alveolar hyperventilation: $\downarrow CO_2$ (hypocarbia, hypocapnia)

Characteristics of HCO_3^-

Normal: 22–26 mEq/L
Metabolic/nonrespiratory parameter
Regulated by the kidneys
Think of HCO_3^- as a base

Normal Arterial and Venous Blood Gas Values

Arterial

pH	7.35–7.45
$Paco_2$	35–45 mm Hg
HCO_3^-	22–26 mEq/L
Pao_2	80–100 mm Hg
Sao_2	>95%
Base excess	− 2 to +2

Venous

pH	7.30–7.40
$P\bar{v}co_2$	46 mm Hg
HCO_3^-	22–26 mEq/L
$P\bar{v}o_2$	40 mm Hg
$S\bar{v}o_2$	70–76%

*Values at sea level.

Compensatory Responses in Acid–Base Disorders

PRIMARY DISORDER	PRIMARY ABNORMALITY	COMPENSATORY RESPONSE	EXPECTED COMPENSATION
Metabolic acidosis	$\downarrow HCO_3^-$ $\downarrow pH$	$\downarrow PaCO_2$	$\Delta PaCO_2 = 1.2 \times \Delta HCO_3^-$
Metabolic alkalosis	$\uparrow HCO_3^-$ $\uparrow pH$	$\uparrow PaCO_2$	$\Delta PaCO_2 = 0.7 \times \Delta HCO_3^-$
Respiratory acidosis			
Acute	$\uparrow PaCO_2$ $\downarrow pH$	$\uparrow HCO_3^-$	$\Delta HCO_3^- = 0.1 \times \Delta PaCO_2$
Chronic	$\uparrow PaCO_2$ $\downarrow pH$	$\uparrow\uparrow HCO_3^-$	$\Delta HCO_3^- = 0.35 \times \Delta PaCO_2$
Respiratory alkalosis			
Acute	$\downarrow PaCO_2$ $\uparrow pH$	$\downarrow HCO_3^-$	$\Delta HCO_3^- = 0.2 \times \Delta PaCO_2$
Chronic	$\downarrow PaCO_2$ Normal to $\uparrow pH$	$\downarrow\downarrow HCO_3^-$	$\Delta HCO_3^- = 0.5 \times \Delta PaCO_2$

Note: $\Delta PaCO_2$ and ΔHCO_3^- are the changes in concentration from normal. $PaCO_2$ is 38–42 mm Hg. HCO_3^- is 24–28 mEq/L. Double arrows indicate a profound change.

From Dantzker DR, MacIntyre NR, Bakow ED: Comprehensive Respiratory Care. Philadelphia, WB Saunders Co, 1995.

Examples of Acute and Chronic/Compensated Respiratory Acidosis and Alkalosis

DISORDER	COMPENSATORY RESPONSE	EXAMPLES	
		Acute	Chronic or Compensated
Respiratory acidosis $\uparrow CO_2$ (>45 mm Hg) $\downarrow pH$ (<7.35)	Hypoventilation; decreased effective alveolar ventilation; reduced CO_2 elimination	pH 7.27 Pco_2 56 HCO_3^- 24	pH 7.36 Pco_2 55 HCO_3^- 39
Respiratory alkalosis $\downarrow CO_2$ (<35 mm Hg) $\uparrow pH$ (>7.45)	Hyperventilation; increased effective alveolar ventilation; excessive CO_2 elimination	pH 7.58 Pco_2 18 HCO_3^- 24	pH 7.49 Pco_2 30 HCO_3^- 21

Examples of Acute and Chronic/Compensatory Metabolic Acidosis and Alkalosis

DISORDER	CAUSE	EXAMPLES	
		Acute	Chronic or Compensated
Metabolic acidosis ↓ HCO_3^- (< 22 mEq/L) ↓ pH (<7.35)	Excessive loss of HCO_3^- or excessive load of acid in the body	pH 7.11 $PaCO_2$ 40 HCO_3^- 12	pH 7.40* $PaCO_2$ 20 HCO_3^- 12
Metabolic alkalosis ↑ HCO_3^- (> 26 mEq/L) ↑ pH (7.45)	Gain of HCO_3^- or excessive loss of acid from the body	pH 7.57 $PaCO_2$ 40 HCO_3^- 36	pH 7.40 $PaCO_2$ 60 HCO_3^- 36

*If the metabolic acidosis is severe, the lungs may not be able to blow off enough CO_2 to compensate. In metabolic acidosis, the body does not compensate fully to return the pH back to 7.40.

Values That May Require Immediate Therapeutic Intervention

pH	<	7.20 pH U
pH	>	7.60 pH U
P_{CO_2}	>	65 mm Hg*
P_{O_2}	<	50 mm Hg

Note: Clinicians should remember to interpret all blood gas values collectively and with regard to the patient's underlying condition because an accurate diagnosis is seldom dependent on a single measured parameter.

*Only in cases with a marked decrease in pH; check HCO_3^- to see if renal compensation has occurred.

Adapted from Burton GG, Hodgkin JE, Ward JJ: Respiratory Care: A Guide to Clinical Practice, 4th ed. Philadelphia, Lippincott-Raven, 1997.

Steps in the Interpretation of an Acid–Base Disorder

Acid–Base Status

1. Evaluate the pH. Is it normal (7.35–7.45), low (<7.35, acidemia), or high (>7.45, alkalemia)?
2. Evaluate the P_{CO_2}. Is it normal (35–45 mm Hg), low (<35 mm Hg), or high (>45 mm Hg)?
3. Evaluate the HCO_3^-. Is it normal (22–26 mEq/L), low (<22 mEq/L), or high (>26 mEq/L)?
4. Determine the primary disorder. Is it respiratory or metabolic (nonrespiratory)?
5. Determine if compensation is present. Is the secondary parameter trending in the same direction as the primary parameter?

Disorder	pH	Primary	Compensation
Respiratory acidosis	↓	↑ CO_2	↑ HCO_3^-
Respiratory alkalosis	↑	↓ CO_2	↓ HCO_3^-
Metabolic acidosis	↓	↓ HCO_3^-	↓ CO_2
Metabolic alkalosis	↑	↑ HCO_3^-	↑ CO_2

6. Compare with previous arterial blood gas level.

Algorithm for Interpretation of Blood Gases

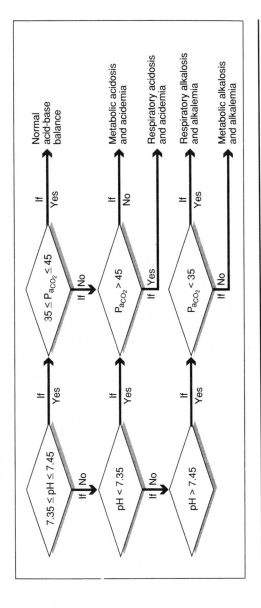

From Cherniak RM: Pulmonary Function Testing, 2nd ec. Philadelphia, WB Saunders Co., 1992, p. 244.

Examples of Arterial Blood Gas Results and Clinical Situations

CLINICAL SITUATION	pH	$Paco_2$	HCO_3^-	Pao_2
			RESULTS	
Acute alveolar hyperventilation with hypoxemia	7.54	29	21	63
Acute ventilatory failure with hypoxemia	7.15	91	28	57
Chronic ventilatory failure with hypoxemia	7.38	88	33	62
Acute alveolar hyperventilation superimposed on chronic ventilatory failure	7.54	57	29	53
Acute ventilatory failure superimposed on chronic ventilatory failure	7.18	103	39	46

From Burton GG, Hodgkin JE, Ward JJ: Respiratory Care: A Guide to Clinical Practice, 4th ed. Philadelphia, Lippincott-Raven, 1997.

Physiologic Effects of Hypoxemia and Signs and Symptoms

Physiologic Effects

> Pulmonary vasoconstriction
> Altered CNS function
> Anaerobic metabolism

Signs and Symptoms

> Mild to moderate hypoxia
>> Tachypnea
>> Hyperventilation
>> Dyspnea
>> Tachycardia
>> Mild hypertension
>> Peripheral vasoconstriction
>> Mild changes in intellectual function
>> Headache
>> Restlessness
> Severe hypoxia
>> Tachypnea
>> Hyperventilation
>> Dyspnea
>> Cyanosis
>> Early-stage tachycardia, leading to bradycardia and dysrhythmias
>> Early-stage hypertension, leading to hypotension
>> Somnolence
>> Confusion
>> Loss of coordination

Measurements of Oxygenation

OXYGENATION MEASUREMENT	DEFINITION	NORMAL RANGE OR VALUES
PaO_2	Partial pressure of oxygen in arterial blood	80–100 mm Hg
SaO_2	Percentage of saturation of hemoglobin with oxygen in arterial blood	>95%
A–aO_2 gradient	Oxygen pressure difference between alveoli and arterial blood; also written as $P(A–a)O_2$ and $A–aDO_2$	5–20 mm Hg
CaO_2	Content of oxygen in arterial blood expressed as milliliters per 100 mL blood or volume %	16–20 mL/100 mL blood
$\dot{Q}_S/\dot{Q}_T$	Shunted cardiac output (L/min) divided by total cardiac output (L/min), expressed as a percentage	3–5%
$P\bar{v}O_2$	Partial pressure of oxygen in mixed venous blood drawn from a pulmonary artery catheter	35–40 mm Hg
$S\bar{v}O_2$	Percent saturation of hemoglobin with oxygen in mixed venous blood	70–76%
$C(a–\bar{v})O_2$	Difference in oxygen content between arterial blood and mixed venous blood, expressed in milliliters per 100 mL blood; also written as $CaO_2 – C\bar{v}O_2$ (volume %)	3.5–5 mL/100 mL blood

From Kersten LD: Comprehensive Respiratory Nursing, Philadelphia, WB Saunders Co., 1989.

Comparison of Normal and Reduced Hemoglobin (Hgb) Levels on Arterial Oxygen Content

	NORMAL VOLUME OF HEMOGLOBIN (15 g/dL)	REDUCED VOLUME OF HEMOGLOBIN (10 g/dL)
O_2 content of Hgb	19.5 vol %	13 vol %
(Hgb $\times$ 1.34) $\times$ % saturation	$(15 \times 1.34) \times 97.5\%$	$(10 \times 1.34) \times 97.5\%$
Dissolved oxygen	0.3 vol % (100 mm Hg $\times$ 0.003)	0.3 vol %
Total oxygen content	19.8 vol %	13.3 vol %

Adapted from Harper RW: A Guide to Respiratory Care. Philadelphia, Lippincott-Raven, 1981.

Normal Adult Values for Complete Blood Count

TEST	NORMAL VALUES
Red blood cell count	
Men	$4.6–6.2 \times 10^6/mm^3$
Women	$4.2–5.4 \times 10^6/mm^3$
Hemoglobin	
Men	13.5–16.5 g/dL
Women	12.0–15.0 g/dL
Hematocrit	
Men	40–54%
Women	38–47%
White blood cell count	$4500–11,500/mm^3$
Differential of white blood cells	
Segmented neutrophils	40–75%
Bands	0–6%
Eosinophils	0–6%
Basophils	0–1%
Lymphocytes	20–45%
Monocytes	2–10%
Platelet count	$150,000–400,000/mm^3$

From Burton GG, Hodgkin JE, Ward JJ: Respiratory Care: A Guide to Clinical Practice, 4th ed. Philadelphia, Lippincott-Raven, 1997.

Systematic Assessment of Chest Radiography

AREA TO ASSESS	OBSERVATIONS
General	Determine if the film is adequate—all structures of the thoracic cage should be visible Assess for gross abnormality not present on previous film (if available) Compare with previous film if possible
Soft tissues (neck, shoulders, axillary area, breast tissue)	Overall physique of patient (overweight, underweight) Nipple shadows
Trachea	Tracheal deviation Tracheal stenosis Position of endotracheal tube
Bony thorax	Ribs, clavicles, scapulae, spine Symmetry of bony structures Absence of bony structures
Intercostal spaces	Symmetry of intercostal spaces Width of spaces—wider space indicates increased lung volume
Diaphragm	Normal—right diaphragm slightly higher than left due to liver (in upright individual); may not be apparent with portable radiograph Flattened diaphragms (lower than normal) seen in chronic obstructive pulmonary disease due to air trapping
Pleural spaces	Lung tissue should extend out laterally to rib margins
Mediastinum	Assess heart and great vessels
Lung fields	Compare sides for symmetry and equal density Vascular markings should be evident out to lateral rib margins Prominence of vascular markings associated with pulmonary edema Assess for haziness, distribution of different densities in lung parenchyma Assess for infiltrate/haziness, especially in basilar areas Assess for placement of lines, tubes

12

Acute Respiratory Failure

Disease Processes That Cause Failure of Ventilation, Oxygenation, Perfusion, or Oxygen Utilization

SYSTEMS, STRUCTURES, AND CONDITIONS	CAUSES OF RESPIRATORY FAILURE
Central nervous system	Drug overdose
	Pickwickian syndrome
	Cerebrovascular accident
	Ondine's curse
	Cerebral trauma ($\uparrow$ ICP)
	Central sleep apnea
	Tumors
	Myxedema
Peripheral nervous system	Multiple sclerosis
	Poliomyelitis
	Amyotrophic lateral sclerosis
	Guillain–Barré syndrome
	Botulism
	Tetanus
	Drugs
	Spinal cord injury
	Myasthenia gravis
	Electrolyte imbalance
Musculoskeletal and pleural functions	Muscular dystrophy
	Kyphoscoliosis
	Flail chest
	Ankylosing spondylitis
	Morbid obesity
	Restrictive pleural diseases
	Pleural effusion
	Pneumothorax
	Hemothorax
Conducting airways	Epiglottitis
	Laryngotracheitis
	Trauma
	Tracheal stenosis
	Foreign body aspiration
	Tumors
	Asthma
	Bronchospasm

(continued)

Disease Processes That Cause Failure of Ventilation, Oxygenation, Perfusion, or Oxygen Utilization (continued)

SYSTEMS, STRUCTURES, AND CONDITIONS	CAUSES OF RESPIRATORY FAILURE
Lungs	COPD
	Cystic fibrosis
	Pneumonia
	Pulmonary emboli
	Aspiration
	Inhaled toxins
	Pulmonary edema
	ARDS
	Interstitial lung disease
	Near drowning
	Inhaled toxins
	Trauma
	Radiation pneumonitis
	Oxygen toxicity
Nonpulmonary conditions	Sepsis
	MI
	Eclampsia
	Anaphylaxis
	Shock
	DIC
	Fat embolism
	SIRS

COPD, chronic obstructive pulmonary disease; ARDS, adult respiratory distress syndrome; MI, myocardial infarction; DIC, disseminated intravascular coagulopathy; SIRS, systemic inflammatory response syndrome; ICP, intracranial pressure.

Patient Factors Influencing Arterial Blood Gas Values

PATIENT FACTORS	Pao_2 NORMS ON ROOM AIR	$Paco_2$ NORMS
Newborn infants	40–70 mm Hg	32–41 mm Hg
Children and adults	80–100 mm Hg	35–45 mm Hg
Elderly adults (> 60 years)	60–80 mm Hg ($103.5 - [0.42 \times age] \pm 4$)	
High altitudes	↓	Normal
Chronic obstructive pulmonary disease	Low normal	↓

Common Drugs That May Cause Respiratory Depression

DRUG CLASS	DRUGS*
Anesthetic agents	Sufentanil citrate (Sufenta)
	Remifentanil hydrochloride (Ultiva)
	Propofol (Diprivan)
Sedatives	Pentobarbital
	Pentobarbital sodium (Nembutal)
	Secobarbital (Seconal)
	Midazolam hydrochloride (Versed)
	Diazepam (Valium)
Paralytics	Pancuronium bromide (Pavulon)
	Succinylcholine chloride
	Tubocurarine chloride (Tubarine)
Analgesics	Codeine
	Fentanyl (Sublimaze)
	Hydromorphone hydrochloride (Dilaudid)
	Meperidine hydrochloride (Demerol)
	Morphine sulfate
	Oxycodone hydrochloride (Percocet)

*Commonly used drugs only, not an exhaustive listing.

Physical Presentation of Common Pulmonary Problems Leading to Acute Respiratory Failure

DISEASE	INSPECTION	PALPATION	PERCUSSION	AUSCULTATION	DEFINITIVE DIAGNOSIS
Pneumonia	Coughing Tachypnea Nasal flaring Use of accessory muscles Purulent sputum	↑ Tactile fremitus	Dullness	Bronchial breath sounds Crackles	CXR Sputum cultures Fever
Emphysema	Pursed-lip breathing Barrel chest	↓ Chest excursion	Hyperresonance	Crackles Prolonged expiration	CXR Pulmonary function tests
Atelectasis	Tachypnea Anxiety Diaphoresis	↑ Tactile fremitus	Dull	Crackles Diminished at bases	CXR Fever
Pulmonary edema	Tachypnea Anxiety Orthopnea Diaphoresis Copious frothy sputum Distended neck veins	↓ Chest excursion	Normal to dull	Dependent crackles Wheezing S_3, S_4 gallop	CXR Fever

CXR, chest radiograph.

Arterial Blood Gas Assessment of Simple Acid–Base Disorders

	pH (7.35–7.45)	PaCO$_2$ (35–45 mm Hg)	HCO$_3^-$ (22–25 mm Hg)	COMPENSATION	
				Respiratory PaCO$_2$	Metabolic HCO$_3^-$
Respiratory					
Acidosis	↓	↑			↑
Alkalosis	↑	↓			↓
Metabolic					
Acidosis	↓		↓	↓	
Alkalosis	↑		↑	↑	

↑, above normal range; ↓, below normal range.

Normal Versus Abnormal Capnogram

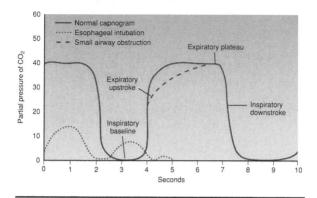

Mixed Acid–Base Disorders

The following are a set of rules to follow when dealing with mixed acid–base disorders:

- A mixed acid–base disorder is present if either the $PaCO_2$ or the HCO_3^- does not follow its predicted value ($\uparrow$ or $\downarrow$) or is not close to its predicted compensatory activity
- Metabolic changes are predictable: For every 10 mEq/L change in HCO_3^-, there should be a 0.15 change in pH
- Respiratory changes are predictable: For every 20 mm Hg increase in $PaCO_2$ above 40 mm Hg, the pH will decrease by 0.10 unit. For every 10 mm Hg decrease in $PaCO_2$ under 40 mm Hg, the pH will increase by 0.10 unit.
- The $PaCO_2$–HCO_3^- relationship is predictable: For every 10 mm Hg $\uparrow$ in $PaCO_2$, there is a corresponding increase of 1 mEq/L of HCO_3^-.

Oxyhemoglobin Dissociation Curve

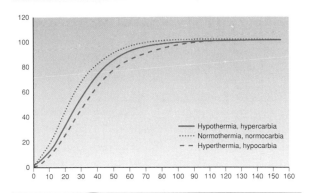

— Hypothermia, hypercarbia
⋯⋯ Normothermia, normocarbia
– – Hyperthermia, hypocarbia

Normal and Abnormal Chest Radiographs

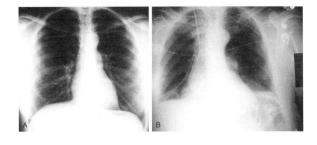

Bedside Pulmonary Measurements

RESPIRATORY PARAMETER	NORMAL VALUE	WEANING PREDICTOR
VOLUMES		
Tidal volume (VT): volume inhaled or exhaled per breath	350–600 mL	>5 mL/kg
Minute ventilation (VE): volume exhaled per minute	4–8 L/min	5–10 L/min
Vital capacity (VC): maximal exhaled volume after a maximal inspiration	60–80 mL/kg* (<20 mL/kg may indicate need for support)	>15 mL/kg (>1,000 mL)
Forced vital capacity (FVC): maximal forceful exhaled volume after a maximal inspiration		
Dead space to tidal volume ratio (VD/VT): the portion of VT that does not participate in gas exchange: $V_D/V_T = PaCO_2 - (P_{ETCO_2} \div PaCO_2)$ (Must be corrected if ventilated)	25–35%, but is position dependent	<60%
AIRWAY PRESSURES		
Peak inspiratory pressure (PIP): maximal pressure during inspiration	Individually trended	>30–33 mL/cm H₂O
Static pressure: pressure required to maintain a delivered VT during a period of no gas flow	Individually trended	

Compliance (C_{dyn}): calculated value indicating volume change per unit of pressure change. Measures lung distensibility:

$C_{dyn} = V_T \div$ (plateau pressure $-$ PEEP)

60–100 mL/cm H_2O (60–80 mL/cm H_2O if ventilated)

Mean airway pressure: average pressure recorded during positive pressure and spontaneous phases of a respiratory cycle

Individually trended

FRACTIONAL GAS CONCENTRATIONS

Exhaled carbon dioxide (P_{ETCO_2}): measures carbon dioxide elimination

Usually 0–5 mm Hg lower than $PaCO_2$

Alveolar to arterial oxygen gradient ($P[A - a] O_2$): indicates gas exchange efficiency:

$PAO_2 = FIO_2 (PBO_2 - PH_2O) - (PaCO_2 \div 0.8)$
$P(A - a)O_2 = PAO_2 - PaO_2$

5–10 mm Hg on room air or 0.4 $\times$ patient's age
<65 mm Hg on 100% O_2

Ratio of arterial to alveolar PO_2 (a/A ratio): proportion of oxygen getting from alveoli to blood, indicates gas exchange efficiency:

$a/A = PaO_2 \div PAO_2$

0.74 in elderly, 0.9 in young adults (90%)

Ratio of arterial partial pressure of oxygen to inspired fractional concentration of oxygen (P/F ratio): assess efficiency of oxygenation, yields a constant value for a given degree of shunting regardless of FIO_2: P/F = $PaO_2 \div FIO_2$

>200

Respiratory index (RI): ratio of alveolar arterial oxygen tension gradient to the arterial partial pressure of oxygen. Measure of efficiency of gas exchange: RI = $P(A - a)O_2 \div PaO_2$

<1.0 (1–5 suggests V/Q imbalance treatable with O_2)

(continued)

Bedside Pulmonary Measurements (continued)

RESPIRATORY PARAMETER	NORMAL VALUE	WEANING PREDICTOR
RESPIRATORY MECHANICS		
Negative inspiratory force or pressure (NIF, NIP): maximum inspiratory pressure the patient is capable of generating against a closed airway	−80 to −100 cm H_2O (60–80 if ventilated)	≤ −30 cm
Maximum voluntary ventilation (MVV): averaged minute ventilation when breathing as deeply and rapidly as possible in 12–15 seconds (measures ventilatory reserve)	120–180 L/min	>Twice V_E
Rapid-shallow breathing index (f/V_T ratio): weaning index: f/V_T = Spontaneous resp. rate (f) ÷ average V_T in liters	Threshold is 100 breaths/min/L >1.8 kg · m/min	100 breaths/min/L 1.6 kg · m/min
Work of breathing index (WOB): measures actual work of breathing		
Oxygen cost of breathing (OCB): difference between whole-body oxygen consumption (Vo) during spontaneous breathing versus that obtained during controlled ventilation: OCB = Vo (spontaneous) − Vo (controlled)	Threshold is 15%	15%
CROP score: combines measures of compliance, rate, oxygenation, and maximum inspiration pressure (MIP): CROP = (C_{dyn} × MIP × a/A) ÷ f	≥18	≥18

*10–15 mL/kg necessary for effective deep breathing and cough.

Respiratory Pharmacology

DRUG	ACTION	SIDE EFFECTS
BRONCHODILATORS*		
Epinephrine (Primatene, Bronkaid, AsthmaHaler)	Adrenergic stimulation; alpha, $beta_1$, $beta_2$ stimulation	Anxiety Tremors Hypertension Tachycardia
Ephedrine sulfate (Ephedrine) Isoproterenol (Isuprel)		Anxiety Tremors Tachycardia Nausea and vomiting Dizziness
Metaproterenol (Alupent) Albuterol (Proventil) Terbutaline sulfate (Brethine, Bricanyl)		

(continued)

Respiratory Pharmacology (continued)

DRUG	ACTION	SIDE EFFECTS
Atropine sulfate	Parasympathetic antagonist	Tachycardia Urinary retention Pupil dilation Dry mouth Slight decrease in mucus clearing
Ipratropium bromide (Atrovent)	Parasympathetic antagonist	
Theophylline, aminophylline (Theo-Dur, Slo-bid)	Inhibit phosphodiesterase, adenosine antagonist	CNS stimulation Diuresis Cardiac stimulation Pulmonary vasodilation
Prostaglandins (PGE_1, PGE_2)	Increase cellular cAMP	Vasodilation
MUCOLYTICS		
N-acetylcysteine (Mucomyst)	Disrupts molecular structure of mucus and lowers viscosity	Nausea Bronchospasm Rhinorrhea Hemoptysis

STEROIDS

Dexamethasone sodium phosphate (Decadron)	Anti-inflammatory, inhibits production and release of histamine, decreases bronchospasm	Hyperglycemia Osteoporosis Increased fat production
Prednisone, prednisolone (Orasone, Deltasone, Meticorten)		Decreased resistance to infection Hypertension
Methylprednisone (Medrol, Solu-Medrol)		
Beclomethasone dipropionate (Vanceril)		Minimal systemic effects Fungal infection in oropharynx or larynx
Flunisolide (AeroBid)		
Triamcinolone acetonide (Aristocort)		

DIURETICS

Furosemide (Lasix)	Loop diuretic	Hypovolemia Hypokalemia Ototoxicity

(continued)

Respiratory Pharmacology (continued)

DRUG	ACTION	SIDE EFFECTS
ANTIBIOTICS/ANTIVIRALS	Treatment of bacterial or viral infections	Ototoxicity Nausea and vomiting Varies
VASOACTIVE DRUGS	Varies: inotropic support, vaso-dilation, vasoconstriction	See chapter 11

*Not all bronchodilators represented.

Data from Scanlan CL, Spearman C, Sheldon RL (eds): *Fundamentals of Respiratory Care.* St. Louis, Mosby–Year Book, 1995.

Airways Most Commonly Used in Acute Respiratory Failure

AIRWAYS	INDICATION	CONTRAINDICATIONS	COMPLICATIONS
Oropharyngeal airway	Unconscious patient Prevent biting during seizures, biting on endotracheal tube	Conscious patient	Gagging Vomiting Discomfort Trauma to palate and oral soft tissues
Nasopharyngeal airway	Unconscious patient Facial injuries Need for frequent nasotracheal suctioning	Sinusitis Closed head injury Basilar skull fracture Coagulopathy present	Discomfort Skin breakdown at nares
Oral endotracheal tubes	Inability to maintain patent airway Emergent intubation Mechanical ventilation	Cautioned with spinal cord injury Cautioned with facial injuries	Greatest risk of self or inadvertent extubation Tube occlusion by biting or trismus Injury to lips, teeth, tongue, palate, and oral soft tissues Retching, gagging, and aspiration Unable to swallow oral secretions Greatest risk of mainstem bronchus intubation Laryngeal or tracheal erosion, necrosis *(continued)*

Airways Most Commonly Used in Acute Respiratory Failure (continued)

AIRWAYS	INDICATION	CONTRAINDICATIONS	COMPLICATIONS

Nasal endotracheal tubes	Inability to maintain patent airway
	Nonemergent intubation
	Mechanical ventilation
	Preferred with cervical spinal cord injury
		Cautioned with facial
		Basilar skull fracture injuries
		Sinusitis
			Greater discomfort during intubation
			Sinusitis
			Epistaxis
			Otitis
			Laryngeal or tracheal erosion, necrosis
			Injury to nares
			Smaller tube required, therefore
			   Greater suctioning difficulty
			   Increased work of breathing

Tracheostomy tubes	Inability to maintain patent airway
	Facial trauma
	Airway obstruction
	Cervical spinal cord injury
	Long-term mechanical ventilation
	   Facilitate weaning
	   Facilitate oral feedings
	   Facilitate communication
		Patients requiring high
		ventilatory pressures
			Hemorrhage
			Infection
			Aspiration
			Voice change
			Mediastinal emphysema
			Tracheoinnominate artery fistula
			Tracheoesophageal fistula
			Tracheal stenosis
			Persistent stoma

Equipment Necessary for Emergent Intubation

- Endotracheal tubes
- Oropharyngeal airway
- Tongue depressor
- 10-mL syringe for cuff inflation
- Plastic-coated malleable stylet
- Magill forceps
- Laryngoscope with curved and straight blades with functioning light
- Water-soluble lubricant
- Spray topical anesthetic
- Manual resuscitation bag and mask
- Oxygen source, flowmeter, and tubing
- Suction equipment, flexible and rigid (Yankauer) suction catheters
- Tape
- Stethoscope
- Gloves, masks, goggles
- Anesthesia induction medications

Supplemental Oxygen Delivery Systems and Clinical Applications

OXYGEN DELIVERY SYSTEM	DESCRIPTION	THEORETIC F_{IO_2}	COMMENTS
Variable performance, low-flow systems:	Provides a portion of inspired gas needs	Varies with patient's minute ventilation	Limited to stable patients
Nasal cannula		0.24–0.44	Limited O_2 delivery for mouth breathers if nasal delivery used
Nasal catheter		0.24–0.60	Flows > 6–8 L/min via nasal cannula are uncomfortable for the patient
Simple face mask		0.40–0.60	Face masks require flows > 5 L/min to avoid CO_2 rebreathing
Partial rebreathing mask		0.65–0.80	
Nonrebreathing mask		0.85–1.0	
Fixed performance, high-flow systems	Meets patient's inspired flow needs	Constant	Best for short-term therapy due to patient discomfort (mask)
Venti-mask		0.24–0.40	May cause mucal drying unless humidity is added
Fixed performance, reservoir systems	Meets the patient's volume needs	Constant	Must be tightly sealed around the patient's face
Leak-free nonrebreathing mask		0.57–0.70	Risk of vomiting and aspiration with tight masks
Air entrainment nebulizers or oxygen blending systems used with		0.50–0.86	Reservoir length on T-piece must be adjusted to prevent rebreathing
T-piece systems			Output flows must meet or exceed inspiratory demands to ensure constant F_{IO_2}
Tracheostomy collar			
Aerosol masks			
Face tents			

Comparison of Various Ventilatory Modes

VENTILATOR MODE	INDICATION	SPECIFIC PATIENT MONITORING*	COMMENTS
CMV	Use for precise control of V_E or $PaCO_2$ (closed head injuries) Perioperative Patients with minimal or no respiratory effort	Level of sedation Asynchronous breathing Acid–base balance PIP Hemodynamic stability	Use with caution for patients with obstructive disorders Patients need sedation to tolerate this mode May worsen hemodynamic status due to positive pressure with each breath Respiratory muscle atrophy
A/C	Perioperative Use to provide complete ventilatory support	Patient comfort PIP Acid–base balance V_E	May worsen air trapping in patients with COPD Hyperventilation problematic if the patient is anxious Respiratory muscle atrophy
SIMV	Provides synchronous partial ventilatory support Provides smooth transitions for weaning	Patient RR PIP Exhaled V_T Spontaneous and ventilator breaths Patient comfort	Improves patient comfort Less respiratory muscle atrophy Increased work of breathing with initiation of spontaneous breaths due to demand flow system

(continued)

Comparison of Various Ventilatory Modes (continued)

VENTILATOR MODE	INDICATION	SPECIFIC PATIENT MONITORING*	COMMENTS
PS	Spontaneous breathing mode May be combined with SIMV Used to unload respiratory muscles (COPD, chronic ventilator patients) Weaning	Exhaled V_T RR Airway cuff leaks (patient will not achieve full V_T) Hemodynamic parameters	Patients find this mode most comfortable Impacts hemodynamic status due to positive pressure Patient retains control over V_T and respiratory pattern V_T can be increased by increasing the pressure support Combine with SIMV if patient has periods of apnea
PC	Full ventilatory support Patients with noncompliant lungs ARDS	Inspiratory pressure level RR Acid–base balance Auto PEEP	Not tolerated without sedation and paralytics Hemodynamic stability often impacted Reduces probability of barotrauma

		PIP should = PC plus set PEEP Cuff pressures Hemodynamics I:E ratio Patient sedation	Requires frequent adjustment of pressures
	Poor oxygenation on volume-cycled ventilators Often used in conjunction with inverse I:E ratio		
MMV	Weaning Often used with PS	RR Acid–base balance	Preset VE does not ensure efficient respiratory pattern Patients usually comfortable Early computerized process
CPAP	Patients with adequate respiratory drive with oxygenation defect Weaning	RR VT Patient comfort Oxygenation and ventilation Assess readiness to extubate	Patient assumes all work of breathing Usually last step prior to extubation May be used without intubation to improve oxygenation

*Patient monitoring and documentation should always include all ventilator settings, pressures, flows, and volumes per unit standards.

A/C, assist/control; ARDS, adult respiratory distress syndrome; CMV, controlled mandatory ventilation; COPD, chronic obstructive pulmonary disease; CPAP, continuous positive airway pressure; I:E, inspiration to expiration ratio; PEEP, positive end-expiratory pressure; PIP, peak inspiratory pressure; PC, pressure control; PS, pressure support; RR, respiratory rate; SIMV, synchronized intermittent mandatory ventilation; VE, minute ventilation; VT, tidal volume.

Ventilator Alarms

VENTILATOR ALARM	USUAL CAUSE	TREATMENT
Oxygen	FIO_2 changed Oxygen analyzer error Oxygen source failure	Reset FIO_2 Recalibrate Reconnect
High pressure (usually set at 10 cm H_2O above average PIP)	Airflow obstruction: mucus, biting, fighting ventilator, water or kinks in tubing	Suction patient Fix kinks in tubing Empty water in tubing Evaluate airway Prevent biting Sedate patient
	Decreased pulmonary compliance: adult respiratory distress syndrome, pneumothorax, hemothorax, pulmonary edema, atelectasis, pneumonia, splinting	Chest tube insertion Suction patient Assess chest radiograph Diureses Increase PEEP Control pain

Low inspiratory pressure (usually set at 5–10 cm H_2O below average PIP)	Ventilator disconnect	Reconnect ventilator to patient
	Air leak	Check cuff patency and replace air in endotracheal tube or tracheostomy cuff if necessary
High exhaled tidal volume or minute ventilation	Increased respiratory rate or tidal volume	Determine and treat cause (anxiety, pain, hypoxemia)
	Inappropriate setting	Reset either alarm, tidal volume or respiratory rate
	Ventilator self-cycling	Decrease sensitivity setting
Apnea (no ventilation for a set time period, 20 sec)	Apnea or respiratory arrest	Provide manual ventilation with bag valve mask
		Determine and treat cause
	Loose connection to exhalation flow sensor	Reconnect
Ventilator inoperative	Loss of electrical power	Manually ventilate, reconnect to power source
	Loss of air or oxygen pressure	Check hoses and reconnect, provide manual ventilation until problem corrected
	Internal hardware malfunction	Manually ventilate and replace ventilator. Send defective ventilator for servicing

PEEP, positive end-expiratory pressure; PIP, peak inspiratory pressure.

Endotracheal Suctioning Technique

Endotracheal suctioning is necessary to remove secretions when a patient is intubated. Nosocomial injury, infection, hypoxia, or airway trauma can be prevented with excellent technique. The following steps must be taken each time you suction a patient:

- Determine need for endotracheal suctioning (breath sounds, coughing, high pressure alarm on ventilator)
- Wash your hands
- Explain procedure to the patient and the family (if present)
- Gather equipment (suction kit, suction tubing to collection canister and gauge, manual resuscitation bag to 100% oxygen, or set ventilator to 100% oxygen)
- Using aseptic technique, open the sterile suctioning kit
- Don sterile gloves
- Determine your nonsterile hand
- Connect suction catheter to suction tubing with nonsterile hand
- Preoxygenate the patient with 100% oxygen. You may use manual breaths via the ventilator or the manual resuscitation bag. Maintain sterility of one hand. It is usually best to have another healthcare provider oxygenate the patient
- Gently insert the suction catheter into the endotracheal tube or tracheostomy tube. Insert until patient coughs. Stop immediately if you feel resistance
- Apply suction only during withdrawal of the catheter
- Hyperoxygenate the patient. Monitor the SpO_2 to avoid hypoxia
- Repeat the suctioning. Note color, consistency, and amount of sputum
- Oxygenate until patient's oxygenation status returns to baseline
- Reassess the patient
- Determine need to send a sputum culture if sputum assessment findings have changed
- Wash your hands
- Document your intervention and assessment findings

The American Association of Respiratory Care* has delineated the following criteria for successful suctioning:

1. Improvement in breath sounds
2. Decreased peak inspiratory pressure
3. Decreased airway resistance
4. Increased tidal volume
5. Improvement in arterial blood gas levels or SpO_2

---

*See Ackerman MH, Ecklund MM, Abu-Jumah M: A review of normal saline instillation: Implications for practice. Dimensions Crit Care Nurs 15:31–38, 1996.

Conditions That Hinder Ventilatory Weaning

CONDITION	PROBLEM
Neuromuscular disorders Age Malnutrition Electrolyte imbalance Muscle atrophy	Decreased vital capacity
Drug therapy Paralytics Sedation Hypothyroidism	Decreased inspiratory force
Sepsis Fever Overfeeding	Abnormally elevated tidal volume
Abdominal distension Pain Anxiety Malpositioning Pneumothorax Hemothorax	Inadequate tidal volume
Pulmonary embolism Emphysema Acute respiratory distress syndrome	Increased dead space
Small endotracheal tube	Increased work of breathing
Auto positive end-expiratory pressure Ventilation circuitry	
Atelectasis Pulmonary embolism Pneumonia Pulmonary edema Bronchospasm	V/Q mismatch

13

Acute Respiratory Distress Syndrome

Recommended Criteria for Acute Lung Injury (ALI) and Acute Respiratory Distress Syndrome (ARDS)

	TIMING	OXYGENATION (Pao_2/Fio_2)	CHEST RADIOGRAPH	WEDGE PRESSURE
ALI	Acute onset	$Pao_2/Fio_2 < 300$ mm Hg regardless of PEEP	Bilateral infiltrates	<18 mm Hg when measured or no clinical evidence of left atrial hypertension
ARDS	Acute onset	$Pao_2/Fio_2 < 200$ mm Hg regardless of PEEP	Bilateral infiltrates	<18 mm Hg when measured or no clinical evidence of left atrial hypertension

PEEP, positive end-expiratory pressure.

Adapted from Bernard G, Artigas A, Brigham K, et al: The American–European consensus conference on ARDS. Am Rev Respir Dis 149:818–824, 1994.

Triggering Events for Acute Lung Injury, Acute Respiratory Distress Syndrome, or Systemic Inflammatory Response

DIRECT PULMONARY INSULTS	INDIRECT PULMONARY INSULTS
Aspiration of gastrointestinal contents	Sepsis
Near drowning	Severe pancreatitis
Inhalation of toxic substances (pesticides, smoke)	Multiple trauma
Inhalation of drugs (cocaine)	Burns
Diffuse pneumonia (bacterial or viral)	Shock
Pulmonary contusion	Cardiopulmonary bypass
Pulmonary embolism	Multiple blood transfusions
End-stage chronic respiratory disease	Neurogenic states
Chronic obstructive pulmonary disease	Nonpulmonary systemic disease
Cystic fibrosis	Anaphylaxis
Oxygen toxicity	Eclampsia
	Diseases of tissue necrosis
	Disseminated intravascular coagulation

Pathophysiologic Progression of Acute Respiratory Distress Syndrome

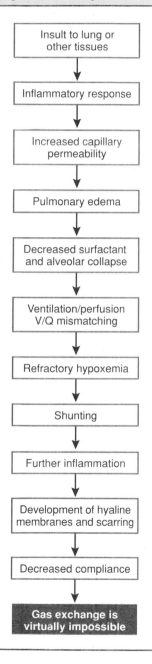

Insult to lung or other tissues

↓

Inflammatory response

↓

Increased capillary permeability

↓

Pulmonary edema

↓

Decreased surfactant and alveolar collapse

↓

Ventilation/perfusion V/Q mismatching

↓

Refractory hypoxemia

↓

Shunting

↓

Further inflammation

↓

Development of hyaline membranes and scarring

↓

Decreased compliance

↓

Gas exchange is virtually impossible

Stages of Acute Respiratory Distress Syndrome (ARDS)

STAGE	MANIFESTATIONS
First	Early exudative phase or acute ARDS. This is manifested by alveolar edema with fibrin and leukocyte debris, damage to type I pneumocytes and endothelial cells
Second	Proliferative phase or subacute ARDS. This is manifested by persistent capillary endothelial damage, type II cell proliferation, and the beginning of squamous transformation
Third	Fibroproliferative phase of chronic ARDS. This is manifested by thickening of the interstitium by an increased number of type II cells and fibrosis

Lung Injury Score

COMPONENT	RANGES	VALUE*
Chest radiograph score	No alveolar consolidation	0
	Alveolar consolidation confined to 1 quadrant	1
	Alveolar consolidation confined to 2 quadrants	2
	Alveolar consolidation confined to 3 quadrants	3
	Alveolar consolidation in all 4 quadrants	4
Hypoxemia score	PaO_2/FiO_2 >300	0
	PaO_2/FiO_2 225–299	1
	PaO_2/FiO_2 175–224	2
	PaO_2/FiO_2 100–174	3
	PaO_2/FiO_2 <100	4
Positive end-expiratory pressure (PEEP) score (when available)	PEEP >5 cm H_2O	0
	PEEP 6–8 cm H_2O	1
	PEEP 9–11 cm H_2O	2
	PEEP 12–14 cm H_2O	3
	PEEP >15 cm H_2O	4

(continued)

Lung Injury Score (continued)

COMPONENT	RANGES	VALUE*
Compliance score (when available)	Compliance >80 mL/cm H_2O	0
	Compliance >50–79 mL/cm H_2O	1
	Compliance >40–59 mL/cm H_2O	2
	Compliance >20–39 mL/cm H_2O	3
	Compliance <19 mL/cm H_2O	4
Total score	No lung injury	0
	Mild to moderate lung injury	0.1–2.5
	Severe lung injury (acute respiratory distress syndrome)	>2.5

*The final value is obtained by dividing the aggregate sum by the number of components that were used.
From Murray J, Matthay M, Luce J, Flick M: An expanded definition of the adult respiratory distress syndrome. Am Rev Respir Dis 138:720–723, 1988.

Pathophysiology of Acute Respiratory Distress Syndrome (ARDS) and Related Treatments

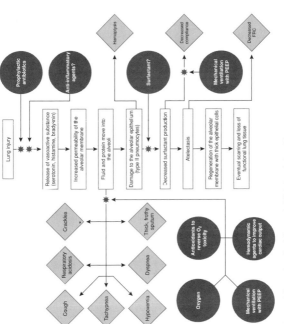

Items noted with a question mark are being researched. Their outcome looks promising.

Recommendations for Administration of Nitric Oxide

1. Atmospheric levels should be controlled by measuring exhaled nitric oxide and nitrogen dioxide levels
2. Methemoglobin levels should be measured routinely
3. Pulse oximetry readings must be watched more closely
4. Delivery must be continuous, and disconnections should be avoided
   Closed-circuit suction systems should be utilized
5. Nitric oxide needs to be weaned slowly, or a rebound pulmonary hypertension may occur
6. Staff, patients, and significant others should be informed of the risk of exposure to nitric oxide
7. Administration of nitric oxide must comply with local environmental pollutant levels, and air quality surveys may be required

Woodrow P: Nitric oxide: Some nursing implications. Intensive Crit Care Nurs 13:87–92, 1997.

Recommendations for Using High Levels of Positive End–Expiratory Pressure (PEEP)

1. Titrate the PEEP in increments of 2–3 cm H_2O until you achieve a level of reduced shunting or approximately 20% or less
2. Maintain an FIO_2 of 40% or less
3. Use tidal volumes of 10–15 mL/kg
4. Use pressure support ventilation to enhance spontaneous breathing
5. Use continuous hemodynamic monitoring (PA line) to monitor for side effects of PEEP and to calculate oxygen transport
6. Treat the hemodynamic compromise of PEEP with blood, fluids, and inotropic infusions as needed

Safcasak K, Nelson L: High-level positive end expiratory pressure management in the surgical patient with acute respiratory distress syndrome. AACN Clin Iss 7(4):482–494, 1996.

14

Pulmonary Embolism

Origins of Pulmonary Emboli

EMBOLISM	ORIGIN
Deep vein thrombosis	Venous stasis Hypercoagulability Vein wall damage
Fat embolism	Fracture of long bones Orthopedic surgery Sternal splitting
Air embolism	IV catheters Trauma: Open chest wounds Diagnostic procedures Surgery: Cardiovascular, abdominal, neurologic Decompression
Amniotic embolism	Amniotic fluid or sac Fluid clots Placental/embryonic tissue
Septic embolism	Massive infection Endocarditis Implanted devices
Tumor embolism	Malignant cells
Right heart embolism	Atrial clots, atrial fibrillation Ventricular clots Prosthetic valve debris Central line/port clots Dialysis Extracorporeal perfusion Valvular calcium
Foreign materials	IV catheters or pulmonary artery/intra-aortic balloon pump balloons Deliberate injection IV drug abuse Non-IV drugs given IV Missiles or bullets Parasitic infestation

Etiology of Deep Vein Thrombosis

LOCATION OF DISORDER	CAUSES
VEIN WALL	IV catheters, sheaths, ports, or shunts
	Inflammation around vein
	Infection around vein
	Varicose veins
	Long-term IV drug abuse
	Direct vessel trauma
	Prior thrombophlebitis
	Post-thrombotic syndrome
	Mechanical manipulation
	Autoimmune disorders
	Major body burns
	Prolonged standing or sitting
	Atherosclerosis
	Familial hyperlipidemias
	Blood type A
	Sports or occupational stress thrombosis
BLOOD	Hyperviscosity
	Dehydration
	Polycythemia
	Surgery
	Trauma or fractures
	Pregnancy and childbirth
	Oral contraceptive use
	Estrogen therapy
	Autoimmune disorders: lupus erythematosus, ulcerative colitis, AIDS, Behçet's syndrome
	Cancer
	Deficient anticoagulation factors: proteins C and S, heparin cofactor II, antithrombin III
	Excessive coagulation factors: fibrinogen, prothrombin, disorder of plasminogen activators
	Irrigation of clotted IVs
	Warfarin-induced hypercoagulability in in first few days of therapy
	Heparin-induced thrombocytopenia
	Hemolytic anemia
BLOOD FLOW	Prolonged bed rest
	Restricted leg activity
	Dependent leg position
	Venous compression
	Diabetes
	Obesity
	Sickle cell anemia
	Prolonged surgery

(continued)

Etiology of Deep Vein Thrombosis (continued)

LOCATION OF DISORDER	CAUSES
BLOOD FLOW (continued)	Peripheral vascular disease
	Low-flow states
	Congestive heart failure
	Myocardial infarction
	Dysrhythmias
	Shock
	Impaired right atrial emptying with atrial fibrillation
	Invasive devices: ports, intra-aortic balloon pumps, IV catheters, pacemakers
	Thoracic outlet syndrome

Deep vein thrombosis can occur with disorders associated with abnormalities in the vein wall due to inflammation, hypercoagulability of the blood, and venous stasis. Additionally, these conditions are risk factors in the development of pulmonary embolism.

Hemodynamic Profile of Severe Pulmonary Embolism

HEMODYNAMIC VALUE	FINDING
Arterial pressure	Normal
	Decreased (with cor pulmonale)
Systemic vascular resistance	Increased
Peripheral vascular resistance	Increased
Central venous pressure/right atrial pressure	Increased
Pulmonary artery diastolic/ pulmonary artery systolic pressure	Increased
Pulmonary artery occlusive pressure	Normal
	Decreased
	Increased (with coexisting left ventricular dysfunction)
Pulmonary artery diastolic/ pulmonary artery occlusive pressure gradient	Widened
Cardiac output/cardiac index	Decreased
Mixed venous oxygen saturation	Decreased

Signs and Symptoms of Confirmed Pulmonary Embolus

SYMPTOMS	PERCENTAGE (%)	PHYSICAL SIGNS	PERCENTAGE (%)
Dyspnea	79.4	General signs	
Chest pain	64.9	Fever	53.6
Apprehension	63.0	Pale	27.8
Sudden dyspnea	58.8	Cyanosis	17.5
Sweating	41.2	Cardiovascular signs	
Dyspnea and chest pain	40.0	Tachycardia >100/min	41.2
Cough	39.2	Increased S_2	40.2
Palpitations	30.9	Hypotension	23.7
Pleuritic chest pain	27.8	Pulmonary artery systolic murmur	22.7
Altered mental status	25.0	Respiratory signs	
Progressive dyspnea	20.6	Breathing rate ≥25/min	58.8
Hemoptysis	13.4	Reduced diaphragm motion	41.2
Syncope	11.3	Decreased breath sounds	38.1
Crushing substernal pain	4.1	Crackles	23.7
		Pleural friction	22.7

FDA-Approved Thrombolytic Regimens for Pulmonary Embolism*

Streptokinase: 250,000 IU as loading dose over 30 min, followed by 100,000 IU/hr for 24–72 hr (approved in 1977)

Urokinase: 4400 IU/kg as loading dose over 10 min, followed by 4400 IU/kg/hr for 12–24 hr (approved in 1978)

Recombinant tissue plasminogen activator: 100 mg continuous infusion over 2 hr (approved in 1990)

*Does not reflect current front-loading administration practices.

Risk Factors for Developing a Pneumothorax

TYPE OF PNEUMOTHORAX	RISK FACTORS
SPONTANEOUS	Bleb or bulla
	Emphysema
	AIDS
	Cystic fibrosis
	Tuberculosis
	Necrotizing pneumonia
	Malignancy
	Barotrauma/positive end-expiratory pressure
	Mechanical ventilation
	Chest tube occlusion
	Chest tube malfunction
	High altitudes
	Decompression diving injuries
	Ankylosing spondylitis
	Lymphangial myxomatosis
	Cocaine use
	Menstruation
TRAUMATIC	Chest surgery
	Insertion of central line
	Thoracentesis
	Gunshot wound
	Knife wound
	Penetrating foreign object
	Falls
	Motor vehicle accidents
	Blunt chest trauma
	Fractured rib

Assessment of the Patient With Chest Tubes

Patient Assessment and Care

1. Assessment should be made at least every 4 hrs
2. Auscultate breath sounds
3. Note respiratory rate, quality, and depth
4. Monitor pulse oximetry
5. Assess for asymmetric chest excursion, hyper-resonance, cyanosis, dyspnea, and decreased or absent breath sounds (which may indicate pneumothorax)
6. Assess for sudden sharp chest pain, anxiety, severe dyspnea, tachycardia, hypotension, dysrhythmias, tracheal deviation to the unaffected side, or neck vein distention (which may indicate tension pneumothorax)
7. Percuss chest for dullness/flatness (which may indicate hemothorax or pleural effusion)
8. Palpate around chest, neck, axilla, and back for subcutaneous emphysema
9. Instruct patient to cough, breathe deeply, and use incentive spirometry every 2 hr
10. Ensure dressing is airtight, clean, dry, and covered with tape

Tubing Assessment and Care

1. Check chest tube to make sure it is secured to the chest
2. Tighten and secure all chest drainage system connections
3. Tighten caps on bottle setups
4. Keep tubing free of kinks, looping, and obstructions to allow free flow of drainage
5. Always keep 2 clamps with the chest tube drainage system
6. Chest tubes should only be clamped under the following circumstances: when physician orders, to change a bottle, if the bottle breaks, or if tubing becomes disconnected from the system for any reason

Drainage System Assessment and Care

1. Keep drainage system below level of patient's chest
2. Stabilize system to prevent tipping or breakage

(continued)

Assessment of the Patient
With Chest Tubes (continued)

3. Assess for fluctuation of drainage in glass straw of bottle setup or in the underwater-seal chamber of disposable system
4. Document the amount, color, and consistency of chest drainage
5. Mark the level of drainage on the tape secured to the bottle or disposable system with the date and time every shift
6. Ensure water seal is intact on a bottle setup by checking that the glass straw extends into the water half an inch and on a disposable system by assessing that the fluid level in the water-seal chamber is at the proper fluid line level
7. Assess for air leaks in the patient and the drainage system

Suction Assessment and Care

1. If chest tube is to be to gravity drainage with no suction, do not clamp the air vent. Remember: no suction, no clamp
2. If bottle setup is to use suction, connect it to a suction machine with an adjustable centimeter suction dial that comes with one or two additional bottles. Clamp off the extra air vent tubing, turn the machine on, and adjust the dial until the ordered amount of suction is indicated
3. If disposable system is to use suction, connect it to low continuous wall suction. The centimeters of suction ordered are adjusted by adding sterile water to the appropriate level in the suction control chamber. Turn the control stopcock to allow gentle bubbling in the suction control chamber and gentle rolling of the small ball in the water-seal chamber
4. If a bottle system is to be converted from suction to gravity drainage, turn off the suction machine, disconnect the tube from the collection bottle of the suction machine, and leave the air vent unclamped. If it is a disposable system, turn off the wall suction, disconnect the tube at the level of the stopcock, and keep the stopcock in the open position

Assessing for Air Leaks

1. If there is continuous bubbling in the bottle setup glass straw or in the disposable water-seal chamber, you have a leak in the system and must clamp and unclamp the tubing in a systematic fashion to determine the source of the leak

2. Never clamp a chest tube for more than 1–2 mins, as this places the patient at risk for tension pneumothorax. Clamping to determine air leaks should not take more than 5–10 seconds

3. Clamp tubing near insertion site and have the patient take several deep breaths while observing the glass straw of a bottle setup or the water-seal chamber of a disposable system for cessation of continuous bubbling. If bubbling stops, the air leak is at the chest tube insertion site or inside the patient. Unclamp the chest tube, and redress and seal the insertion site with occlusive Vaseline gauze, a large dressing, and tape. If bubbling continues, the leak may be inside the patient. If patient is symptomatic, contact the physician immediately

4. If the bubbling continues, clamp the tubing at 4–6 inch increments and check the water seal for continuous bubbling. When the bubbling stops, the leak is between the present position and the previous position. Tighten all connections in this area, and try to seal a leak in the tube with tape

5. If bubbling continues after checking the entire length of the tubing, the leak is in the drainage collection system itself. Prepare an additional drainage collection system according to manufacturer instructions. Clamp the chest tube, disconnect from the old system, reconnect to the new system, and unclamp the chest tube. Reassess again for air leaks

Managing Problems of Chest Tube Drainage

CHEST DRAINAGE PROBLEM	NURSING INTERVENTION
Chest tube is dislodged	Immediately place gloved hand over insertion site and call for assistance
	Secure occlusive Vaseline dressing and dry gauze dressing over insertion site with tape
	Reassess patient and notify physician
Drainage system breaks, or tubing pulls apart and is contaminated	Clamp chest tube
	Irrigate contaminated tubing with sterile water or saline and place end of tubing into sterile solution at least 2–4 cm below fluid surface
	Stay with patient while another nurse obtains and sets up a new collection system
	Connect new system to chest tube
No fluctuation of fluid in glass straw of bottle setup or water-seal chamber of disposable system during respirations	Reposition patient and have cough and breathe deeply. Assess for respiratory difficulty
	Gently milk or squeeze chest tubing
	Fluctuation will decrease as lung expands
	Fluctuation stops if lung is expanded and sealed

Dramatic increase in chest drainage of 200 mL in 1 hr / 100 mL/hr × 3 hr / 500 mL in 8 hr	Note activity before increase occurred. Dumping of pockets of fluid can occur with position changes Note drainage color, amount, and consistency Assess vital signs for increased pulse rate, orthostatic or dropping blood pressure changes that could indicate acute hemorrhage, and respiratory status Notify physician. Recheck patient every 5–15 min
Continuous bubbling in glass straw of bottle setup or water-seal chamber of disposable system	*Check for air leaks
Abnormal bubbling in suction-control chamber of disposable system	No bubbling; check for obstructions and that suction source is connected and turned on Vigorous bubbling: turn stopcock suction control until slow, gentle bubbling is visible
Too little or too much fluid in water-seal or suction-control chambers of disposable system	Pinch off to suction source to check for level of fluid in suction-control chamber If below required level, add more sterile water or system saline to chamber through resealable diaphragm or with a syringe and needle or through the top filling port If above required level, remove excess fluid with a syringe and needle through resealable diaphragm. *Do not* tip over to remove fluid
Collection system turns over, is placed higher than chest, or tubing is obstructed	Place collection system in proper position Unkink tubing and gently milk if permitted Have patient take some deep breaths and cough

Criteria for Lung Reduction Surgery Candidates

Advanced emphysema
Unhappy with emphysema limitations
Small amount of airway inflammation
Controlled or no active medical problems
No or low-dose systemic steroid use
Active participation in pulmonary rehabilitation
    program
No smoking in past year
Residual volume > 150% predicted
Systolic pulmonary artery pressures < 50 mm Hg

Criteria for Lung Transplantation Candidates

Inclusion Criteria

Forced vital capacity of < 40% predicted
FEV_1 (first second of expiration) < 30% of predicted
Room Air PaO_2 < 60 mm Hg at rest
Predicted survival < 2 years
Major pulmonary complications
Increased antibiotic resistance

Exclusion Criteria

Ongoing infection related to
    AIDS
    Hepatitis B
    Mycobacterium tuberculosis
    Burkholderia cepacia
    Methicillin-resistant *Staphylococcus aureus*
    Aspergillus sp.
    Multiply resistant *Pseudomonas aeruginosa*
Hepatic, renal, or left ventricular failure
Diabetes with severe end-organ failure
Symptomatic osteoporosis
Inability to ambulate
Ventilator dependent
Significant psychiatric disorder

Adapted from Mallory GB, Yankaskas JR: Lung transplantation: Consensus and controversies. In Highlights: Selected Proceedings From the Tenth Annual North American Cystic Fibrosis Conference, October 24–27, 1996, p. 20.

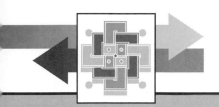

Renal
Disorders

15

Renal Anatomy and Physiology

Gross Structures of the Kidney

Glomerular Pressures and Filtration

Systemic Reactions of Angiotensin II

Alterations in the Renal System Due to Aging

Gross Structures of the Kidney

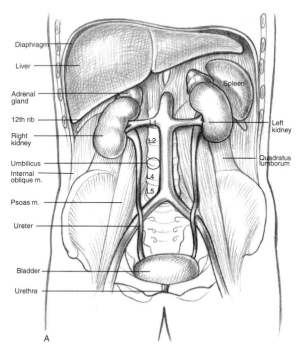

A

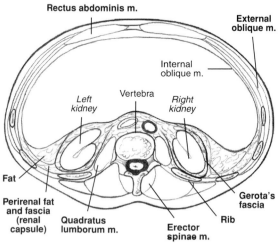

B

(continued)

Gross Structures of the Kidney
(continued)

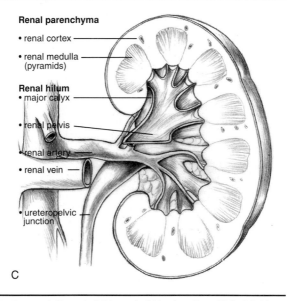

Renal parenchyma
- renal cortex
- renal medulla (pyramids)

Renal hilum
- major calyx
- renal pelvis
- renal artery
- renal vein
- ureteropelvic junction

C

Luckmann J: Saunder's Manual of Nursing Care. Philadelphia, W.B. Saunders, Co., 1997.

Glomerular Pressures and Filtration

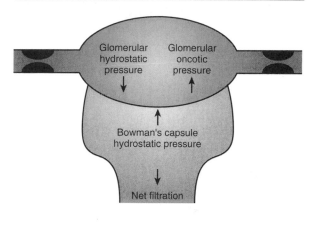

Net filtration pressure (10 mm Hg)	=	Glomerular hydrostatic pressure (60 mm Hg)	−	Bowman's capsule hydrostatic pressure (18 mm Hg)	−	Glomerular oncotic pressure (32 mm Hg)

Redrawn from Guyton A, Hall J: *Textbook of Medical Physiology*, 9th ed. Philadelphia, W.B. Saunders, 1996, p. 322.

Systemic Reactions of Angiotensin II

ACTION	REACTION
PRODUCES PERIPHERAL ARTERIOLAR VASOCONSTRICTION	Causes a rise in systolic and diastolic blood pressures, which increases systolic/diastolic blood pressure and arteriolar vasoconstriction; increases renal blood flow; increases afferent arteriolar blood flow and pressure; increases glomerular pressure; increases or maintains glomerular filtration rate; causes correction or maintenance of renal function
STIMULATES SECRETION OF ALDOSTERONE	Causes reabsorption of water, Na$^+$, Cl$^-$ in distal convoluted tubule, which increases systemic blood pressure; increases renal blood flow; increases or maintains glomerular filtration rate; causes correction or maintenance of renal function
STIMULATES ANTIDIURETIC HORMONE (VASOPRESSIN)	Causes an increase in reabsorption of water in collecting tubule, which increases systemic blood volume and pressures; increases renal blood flow; increases or maintains glomerular filtration rate; causes correction or maintenance of renal function
STIMULATES POSTSYMPATHETIC NEURONS TO RELEASE NOREPINEPHRINE	Causes an increase in vasoconstriction, which increases systemic blood pressure; increases renal blood flow; increases or maintains glomerular filtration rate; causes correction or maintenance of renal function

Alterations in the Renal System Due to Aging

Decreased perception of thirst, resulting in changes in blood volume; in situations of actual shifts in hydration resulting from heat, diarrhea, or decreased food and fluid intake, this alteration may become clinically significant

Renal blood flow decreased, resulting in a decreased glomerular filtration rate. In persons with systemic vascular disease, which may also contribute to decreased renal blood flow (e.g., atherosclerosis, congestive heart failure), this combination may be clinically significant

Decreased renin response to volume loss prevents the aged kidney from increasing renal blood flow and systemic blood pressures through stimulation of the renin-angiotensin system (as previously described)

Both maximum concentration and dilution of urine decrease by the seventh decade of life. These changes add to the aged person's risks of hypo- and hypervolemia in the face of changes in vascular volume. In combination with the altered renin response, these changes make the elderly especially vulnerable to hypotension when fluid losses occur or to overhydration and hyponatremia when vigorous hydration is required

Decreased NH_4^+ (ammonia) secretion also decreases the aged person's ability to maintain or correct a state of metabolic acidosis. This decrease in function may contribute to and exacerbate other acid-base abnormalities

16

Renal Assessment

Drug Elimination in Renal Failure

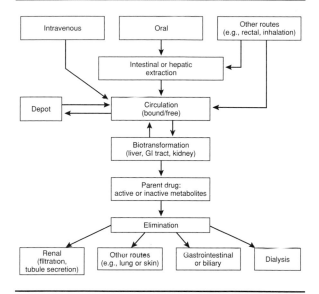

Shuler C, Golper TA, Bennett WM: Prescribing drugs in renal disease. In Brenner BM (ed): Brenner & Rector's The Kidney, vol. 11. Philadelphia, W.B. Saunders Co., 1996, p. 2654.

Common Nail Findings Associated With Renal Disease

BEAU'S LINES   MEES' BANDS   LINDSAY'S NAILS   TERRY'S NAILS

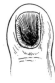 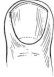

KOILONYCHIA   CLUBBING   PSORIASIS

From Swartz MH: Textbook of Physical Diagnosis: History and Examination, 2nd ed. Philadelphia, W.B. Saunders Co., 1996, p. 76.

Fingernail Assessment

FINDING	CHARACTERISTICS	ETIOLOGY
Beau's lines	Transverse grooves due to sporadic decrease in nail growth	Chronic renal or liver disease
Mees' bands	White transverse marks	Acute renal toxicities from poisonings or acute systemic disease
Lindsay's nails (or half-and-half)	Proximal half of the nail appears whitish; distal portion is reddish or pink	Renal disease
Terry's nails	White nail beds with small area of normal color in distal 1–2 mm border	Low albumin due to cirrhosis or renal disease
Koilonychia (spoon nails)	Nail indented	Iron deficiency anemia, a common finding in patients with renal abnormalities
Clubbing	Broadened upper portion of finger and nail bed	Cardiovascular compromise
Pitted nails	Small pits in surface of nail	Psoriasis

Testing for Pitting Edema of the Lower Extremities

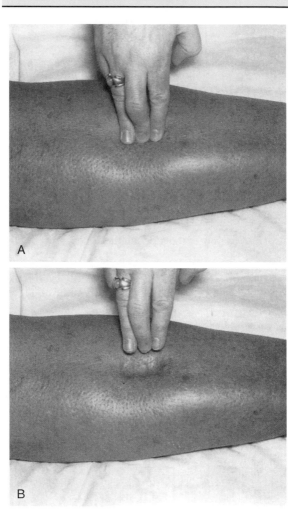

From Swartz MH: Textbook of Physical Diagnosis: History and Examination, 2nd ed. Philadelphia, W.B. Saunders Co., 1996, p. 258.

Technique for Kidney Palpation

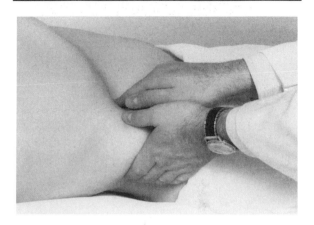

From Swartz MH: Textbook of Physical Diagnosis: History and Examination, 2nd ed. Philadelphia, W.B. Saunders Co., 1996, p. 327.

Technique Used in Assessing Costovertebral Tenderness

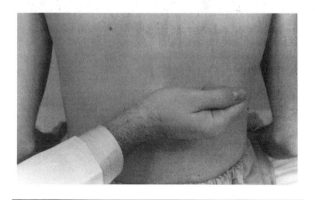

From Swartz MH: Textbook of Physical Diagnosis: History and Examination, 2nd ed. Philadelphia, W.B. Saunders Co., 1996, p. 328.

Electrolyte Disturbances Associated With Acute or Chronic Renal Failure

Hypokalemia or hyperkalemia
Hyponatremia or hypernatremia
Hypocalcemia or hypercalcemia
Hypomagnesemia or hypermagnesemia
Hypochloremia or hyperchloremia
Hypophosphatemia or hyperphosphatemia

17

Renal Laboratory and Diagnostic Tests

Common Blood Assessments Performed and Values Expected With Renal Compromise

BLOOD TEST	NORMAL VALUE	RENAL COMPROMISE
Serum albumin	3.4–4.7 g/dL	Reduced
Blood urea nitrogen	8–20 mg/dL	Elevated
Creatinine	0.6–1.2 mg/dL	Elevated
Serum osmolality	275–293 mOsm/kg H_2O	Elevated or decreased
Hemoglobin	Females: 12.0–15.5 g/dL	Decreased
	Males: 13.6–17.5 g/dL	Decreased
Hematocrit	Females: 35–45%	Decreased
	Males: 39–49%	Decreased
Serum magnesium	1.8–3.0 mg/dL	Decreased or elevated with ingestion of large amounts of magnesium in laxatives
Serum electrolytes		Elevated or decreased

Concentration (mEq/L) of Electrolytes in Various Body Fluids*

FLUID	SODIUM	POTASSIUM	CHLORIDE	BICARBONATE	HYDROGEN
Plasma	135–145	3.5–5.0	98–106	25–29	7.35–7.45
Gastric juices	55–100	10–15	120	5–10	90
Pancreatic juices	145–160	5	65–90	50–80	—
Bile	130–145	5–9	75–100	10–45	—
Ileum	125	10–80	55	60	—
Sweat					
Insensible	8	10	15	—	—
Sensible	10–80	6	5–85	—	—

*Levels may vary depending on the physiologic state of the body.

From White B: Maintaining fluid and electrolyte balance. In Bolander VB (ed.): *Sorenson and Luckmann's Basic Nursing: A Psychophysiologic Approach*, 3rd ed. Philadelphia, W.B. Saunders Co, 1997, p. 294.

Urine Indices Used in the Differential Diagnosis of Prerenal and Intrinsic Renal Azotemia

DIAGNOSTIC INDEX	PRERENAL AZOTEMIA	ISCHEMIC INTRINSIC AZOTEMIA
Fractional excretion of Na^+ (%),* $\dfrac{U_{Na} \times P_{cr}}{P_{Na} \times U_{cr}} \times 100$	<1	>1
Urinary Na^+ concentration (mEq/L)	<10	>20
Urinary creatinine/plasma creatinine ratio	>40	<20
Urinary urea nitrogen/plasma urea nitrogen ratio	>8	<3
Urine specific gravity	>1.018	<1.012
Urine osmolality (mOsm/kg H_2O)	>500	<250
Plasma BUN/creatinine ratio	>20	<10–15
Renal failure index,* $U_{Na}/U_{cr}/P_{cr}$	<1	>1
Urine sediment	Hyaline casts	Muddy brown granular casts

*Most sensitive indices.

BUN, blood urea nitrogen; Na^+, sodium; P_{cr}, plasma creatinine concentration; P_{Na}, plasma Na^+ concentration; U_{cr}, urine creatinine concentration; U_{Na}, urine Na^+ concentration.

From Brady H, Brenner BM, Lieberthal W: Acute renal failure. In Brenner BM (ed): The Kidney, 5th ed., vol. 2. Philadelphia, W.B. Saunders Co, 1997, p. 1227.

Creatinine Clearance

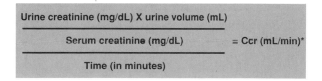

MALES	$\dfrac{(140 - \text{age in years}) \times \text{weight (kg)}}{\text{Serum creatinine (mg/dL)} \times 72} = \text{Creatinine clearance (mL/min)}$
FEMALES	$\dfrac{(140 - \text{age in years}) \times \text{weight (kg)}}{\text{Serum creatinine (mg/dL)} \times 72} \times 0.85 = \text{Creatinine clearance (mL/min)}$

Creatinine Clearance (Ccr) Adjusted by Body Surface Area (BSA)

$$\dfrac{\dfrac{\text{Urine creatinine (mg/dL)} \times \text{urine volume (mL)}}{\text{Serum creatinine (mg/dL)}}}{\text{Time (in minutes)}} = \text{Ccr (mL/min)}^*$$

A more accurate picture of renal function is obtained when the creatinine clearance is adjusted for the patient's body surface area (Ccr = ml/min/1.73 m^2 BSA).

18

Acute Renal Failure

Common Causes of Acute Renal Failure

CATEGORY	CAUSE
PRERENAL	Volume
	Dehydration
	Ischemic
	Hypotensive shock
	Cardiogenic shock
	Septic shock
	Hypoxemia
	Reduced cardiac output
POSTRENAL	Urethral
	Stricture
	Prostatic hypertrophy
	Ureteral
	Fibrosis
	Calculi
	Blood clots
	Bladder
	Neurogenic problems
	Neoplasms
	Obstruction
RENAL	Glomerular
	Acute glomerulonephritis
	Acute cortical necrosis
	Hepatorenal syndrome
	Tubular
	Acute tubular necrosis
	Acute pyelonephritis
	Nephrotoxins
	Heavy metals
	Antibiotics
	Radiographic contrast media
	Anesthetics
	Pigments
	Hemoglobin
	Myoglobin

Differences Between Acute and Chronic Renal Failure

TYPE OF RENAL FAILURE	ONSET	PROGNOSIS	SYMPTOMS	TREATMENT
Acute	Sudden	Reversible	Dramatic; no time for compensation by body, therefore should treat all imbalances	Hemodialysis, peritoneal dialysis, and continuous renal replacement therapy
Chronic	Slow, progressive (3 or more years until end stage)	Irreversible	Gradual; time for body to compensate, therefore may have time before treatment is necessary	Hemodialysis, peritoneal dialysis

Comparison of Laboratory Findings in Prerenal, Postrenal, and Intrinsic Renal Oliguric States

VALUE	PRERENAL	POSTRENAL	INTRINSIC RENAL (ACUTE TUBULAR NECROSIS)
Urine volume	Decreased	May alternate between anuria and polyuria	Anuria <100 mL/24 hr Oliguria 100–400 mL/24 hr Nonoliguria >400 mL/24 hr
Urine osmolality	Increased (>500 mOsm)	Isotonic (≤350 mOsm)	Isotonic (≤350 mOsm)
Urine specific gravity	Increased (>1.020)	Fixed (1.008–1.012)	Fixed (1.008–1.012)
Urine sodium	<20 mEq/L	>40 mEq/L	>40 mEq/L
Fractional excretion of sodium (FE_{Na})*	<1%	>1%	>1%
Urine failure index†	<1%	>1%	>1%
Urine pH	<6.0	>6.0	>6.0
Urine protein	Minimal	Minimal	Increased
Urine sediment	Normal, few casts	Normal, histiocytes and crystals	Granular casts, tubular epithelial cells
Urine/plasma creatinine ratio	>40	<20	<20
Blood urea nitrogen: serum creatinine	>20:1	10–15:1	10–15:1

*Fractional excretion of sodium = U/P sodium ÷ U/P creatinine × 100, where U is urine and P is plasma.

†Renal failure index = U sodium ÷ U/P creatinine, where U is urine and P is plasma.

Adapted from Brezis M, Rosen S, Epstein FH: Acute renal failure. In Brenner BM, Rector FC (eds): *The Kidney*, 4th ed. Philadelphia, W.B. Saunders Co., pp. 993–1061.

Patients at High Risk for Acute Renal Failure

- Hemodynamic instability
- Multiple organ dysfunction
- Trauma victim
- Intravenous hemolysis
- Rhabdomyolysis
- Nephrotoxic agents
- Complicated postoperative course

Electrolyte Imbalances and the Effect on Cardiac Function

ELECTROLYTE	ACTION ON MYOCARDIUM
Hyperkalemia	↓ Contractility ↓ Conduction asystole ECG changes: tall, peaked T wave, disappearance of P wave, widened QRS
Hypokalemia	Dysrhythmias Digoxin toxicity ECG changes: depressed ST segments, flat or inverted T wave, presence of U wave
Hypercalcemia	Enhanced digoxin effect ECG changes: shortened ST segment, increased incidence of heart block, cardiac arrest
Hypocalcemia	Dysrhythmias ECG changes: prolonged ST segment and QT interval
Hyperphosphatemia	ECG changes: prolongation of ST segment
Hypermagnesemia	Bradycardia ECG changes: peaked T waves similar to hyperkalemia Depressed contractility
Hypomagnesemia	Dysrhythmias ECG changes: flat or inverted T waves, possible ST segment depression, prolonged QT interval

Supportive Therapy in Ischemic and Nephrotoxic Acute Tubular Necrosis

PATIENT PROBLEMS	TREATMENT*
Extracellular volume overload	Restriction of salt (2–4 g per day) and water (usually <1 L/day) Diuretics, if responsive (usually loop blockers and thiazide) Dialysis (daily or continuous)
Hyponatremia (dilutional)	Restriction of oral water intake (<1 L/day) Restriction of hypotonic intravenous solutions (including dextrose-containing solutions)
Hyperkalemia	Restriction of dietary potassium intake (20–50 mEq/day) Eliminate potassium supplements and potassium-sparing diuretics Potassium-binding ion-exchange resins (e.g., sodium polystyrene sulfonate) Dialysis; consider low-potassium dialysate Glucose (50 mL 50% dextrose) and insulin (10 U regular) Sodium bicarbonate (usually 50–100 nmol/L) Calcium gluconate (10 mL 10% solution over 5 min)
Metabolic acidosis	Sodium bicarbonate (maintain serum bicarbonate >15 nmol/L, arterial pH >7.2) Dialysis
Hyperphosphatemia	Restriction of dietary phosphate intake (<800 mg/day) Phosphate-binding agents (calcium carbonate, aluminum hydroxide) Dialysis
Hypocalcemia	Calcium carbonate PO (if symptomatic or if sodium bicarbonate to be administered) Calcium gluconate (10–20 mL 10% solution IV; consider if emergency) Dialysis

(continued)

Supportive Therapy in Ischemic and Nephrotoxic Acute Tubular Necrosis (continued)

PATIENT PROBLEMS	TREATMENT*
Hypermagnesemia	Discontinue magnesium-containing antacids Dialysis
Hyperuricemia	Treatment usually not necessary (if serum uric acid < 15 mg/dL) Allopurinol and forced alkaline diuresis if > 30 mg/dL,
Nutrition	High dietary protein (35 to 50 kcal/kg of ideal body weight per day) Enteral and parenteral nutrition
Drug dosage	Adjust doses for glomerular filtration rate (generally < 10 mL/min) Avoid nonsteroidal anti-inflammatory agents, angiotensin-converting enzyme inhibitors, radiocontrast agents, nephrotoxic antibiotics (unless absolute indication)

*These are general guidelines and must be tailored to the needs of individual patients.

Adapted from Anderson RJ: Prevention and Management of Acute Renal Failure. Hosp Pract 28: 61–75, 1993.

Indications for Renal Dialysis

- Uremic syndrome (interfering with activities of daily living)
- Uremic pericarditis
- Volume overload
- Electrolyte imbalances
- Symptomatic metabolic acidosis
- Overdose (drug must be lipid free)

19

Chronic Renal Failure and Renal Transplantation

Treatment of Hyperkalemia

TREATMENT STRATEGY	MECHANISM OF ACTION
IV THERAPY	
Calcium chloride	Stabilizes the irritability of cardiac muscle
Sodium bicarbonate	Improves metabolic acidosis, which alters cell wall potential (potassium moving out of cell is reversed)
50% Glucose plus regular insulin	Transports potassium from extracellular to intracellular compartment
ORAL/RECTAL THERAPY	
Kayexalate (often mixed in liquid sorbitol)	Resin, which exchanges sodium for potassium ion in the gastrointestinal tract; binds the potassium ion for excretion in the feces
	Sorbitol is an inert sugar that stimulates osmotic fluid shift into gastrointestinal tract lumen; creates diarrhea, which enhances quick, efficient potassium loss
EXTRACORPOREAL THERAPY	
Hemodialysis	Moves potassium from blood into dialysate via diffusion
Peritoneal dialysis	Removes potassium from body via dialysate outflow

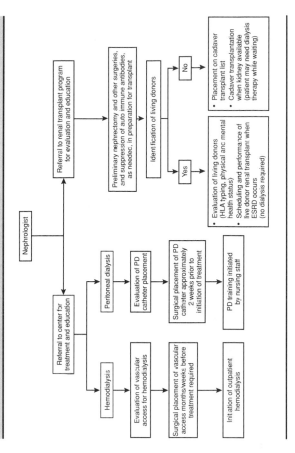

HLA Matching for Donor Compatibility

HLA identities here are represented as numbers to identify possible combinations

MOTHER	FATHER
1 2	3 4

OFFSPRING (CHILDREN)

Sibling 1	Sibling 2	Sibling 3	Sibling 4	Sibling 5
1 3	2 4	2 3	1 4	2 4

Siblings 2 and 5 are HLA identical; sibling 1 is totally dissimilar to siblings 2 and 5; sibling 3 is half-identical to siblings 1, 2, and 5.

Nonrelated donors may be identical, 50% match, 25% match, or totally dissimilar.

Immunosuppressant Therapy After Kidney Transplantation*

DRUG	ACTION	NURSING AND PATIENT IMPLICATIONS
AZATHIOPRINE (IMURAN)	Bone marrow suppression, specifically white blood cells; inhibits the early stages of cell differentiation and proliferation	Useful in preventing rejection but ineffective in treating acute rejection. May be administered intravenously and orally. Major side effect is hepatoxicity
CORTICOSTEROIDS (SOLU-MEDROL, PREDNISONE)	Immunosuppressive effects: interfere with gene transcription and alter cell function (RNA translation, protein synthesis, and secretion of cytokines and proteins); decrease number of circulating lymphocytes; inhibit events associated with T-cell activation; and inhibit early proliferation of B cells Anti-inflammatory effects: inhibit accumulation of leukocytes at site of inflammation; inhibit macrophage function and decrease production of prostaglandins	Used in conjunction with other immunosuppressive drugs. Many short-term and long-term side effects: Cushing's syndrome. Patients may develop adrenal crisis if therapy is withdrawn abruptly (as may be the inadvertent case in patients whose transplanted kidneys have failed. May be given intravenously or orally

(continued)

Immunosuppressant Therapy After Kidney Transplantation* (continued)

DRUG	ACTION	NURSING AND PATIENT IMPLICATIONS
CYCLOSPORINE (SANDIMMUNE, NEORAL)	Inhibits the early activities of T-cell activation, sensitization, and proliferation	Used to prevent acute rejection. Minimal effect on mature cytotoxic T cells, thus cannot reverse acute ejection. Effect on suppression of B cells and chronic rejection is unclear. Can be administered intravenously and orally
TACROLIMUS (PROGRAF)	Inhibits T-lymphocyte activation by binding to intracellular protein and forming a complex that prevents the generation of nuclear material for activated T cells	Effective as rescue or emergency therapy during an episode of acute or chronic rejection. May be reserved for the treatment of these events rather than used as a primary immunosuppressant
ANTITHYMOCYTE GLOBULIN (ATG, ATGAM)	Antibody made from horse serum that binds to T- and B-cell lymphocytes as well as platelets and granulocytes, thus depleting and lysing immunologically active cells and reversing acute rejection episodes	Usually reserved for prophylaxis or induction immediately before or at the time of transplant. Also used for acute graft rejection that does not respond well to corticosteroids. Side effects are similar to those of serum sickness. In addition, patients may become sensitized to the horse serum and may be at risk for an anaphylactic reaction

MURINE MONOCLONAL ANTIBODY (OKT3)	Monoclonal antibody that suppresses T cell mediated rejection by binding to specific regions of the T cell, thus altering T cell recognition of the antigen; blocks killer T cells that are attached to the transplanted kidney and renders them inactive	Used to suppress acute episodes of rejection. Can only be given intravenously and may produce systemic reactions. Allergic reactions, including anaphylaxis, can occur
MYCOPHENOLATE (CELLCEPT)	Suppresses T and B lymphocyte proliferation. Inhibits the enzyme inosine monophosphate dehydrogenase, which is required for protein synthesis	Often used in combination with cyclosporine and corticosteroids to prevent rejection

*Patients on immunosuppressive therapy are at high risk for infections. The nurse should carefully investigate any (even subtle) changes in the patient's status as the usual signs and symptoms of infections may be masked. If the patient requires blood, the blood should be irradiated. Use of invasive lines should be minimized and adherence to aseptic technique absolute.

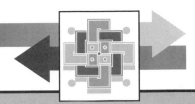

Endocrine
Disorders

20

Endocrine Anatomy and Physiology

Chemical Makeup of Hormones

Steroids	Amino Acid Analogs	Peptides
Product of cholesterol breakdown	Derivative of the amino acid tyrosine	Large proteins or chains of proteins
Adrenal Cortex	**Thyroid**	**Anterior Pituitary**
Glucocorticoids (cortisol)	Thyroxine (T_4)	Adrenocorticotropin
Mineralocorticoids (aldosterone)	Triiodothyronine (T_3)	Growth hormone
Androgens		Follicle-stimulating hormone
		Luteinizing hormone
		Prolactin
		Thyroid-stimulating hormone
		Melanocyte-stimulating hormone
	Adrenal Medulla	**Posterior Pituitary**
Ovaries	Epinephrine	Antidiuretic hormone (vasopressin)
Progesterone	Norepinephrine	Oxytocin
Estrogen		

(continued)

Chemical Makeup of Hormones (continued)

Testes
Testosterone

Placenta
Estrogen
Progesterone

Pancreas
Glucagon
Insulin

Parathyroid
Parathyroid hormone

Thyroid
Calcitonin

Summary of the Effects of Glucocorticoids

TARGET SYSTEM	CONSEQUENCES
Metabolism	Increase in gluconeogenesis Decrease in peripheral glucose uptake Insulin resistance Increase in glycogen synthesis Glycolysis, generally a catabolic process
Connective tissue	Inhibition of fibroblasts, causing loss of collagen, and resulting in thinning of skin Easy bruising Poor wound healing
Bone/calcium metabolism	Inhibition of bone formation by decreasing cell proliferation Inhibition of RNA, protein, and collagen synthesis Stimulation of bone reabsorption, leading to bone loss Stimulation of parathyroid hormone and vitamin D production and its effectiveness Reduction of gastrointestinal absorption of calcium
Growth/development	Inhibition of growth in children, secondary to decreased growth hormone
Hematologic/immune	Reduction in the number of mast cells Stabilization of lysosomal membranes, thus inhibiting release of histamine Decrease in capillary permeability Depression of phagocytosis Decrease of interleukin-1, which causes fever Atrophy of all lymphatic tissue
Cardiovascular	Increase in cardiac output Increase in vascular tone Effects of catecholamines potentiated Regulation of adrenergic receptors Elevation of triglycerides/cholesterol due to an increase in lipolysis

(continued)

Summary of the Effects of Glucocorticoids (continued)

TARGET SYSTEM	CONSEQUENCES
Renal	Increase in glomerular rate with electrolyte imbalances
CNS	Impairments in memory and concentration Insomnia with decreased REM sleep Increased stage II sleep Depression/acute steroid psychosis
Ophthalmologic	Intraocular pressure is thought to vary with the level of cortisol (parallels the circadian rhythm of cortisol) Possible cataract formation
Other hormones	Decrease in thyroid response to thyrotropin-releasing hormone Decrease in T_3 due to a decrease in the conversion of T_4 to T_3 Decrease in the response of testes to gonadotropin-releasing hormone, leading to low testosterone levels Suppression of luteinizing hormone, leading to low levels of estrogen/progesterone and causing amenorrhea and anovulation

21

Endocrine Assessment

Hormonal Activity Suggested
by Clinical Findings

Hormonal Activity Suggested by Clinical Findings

CLINICAL FINDINGS	HORMONAL INFLUENCE
HEMODYNAMIC REGULATION	
Hypertension	↑ Catecholamines; ↑ aldosterone; ↑ ACTH/cortisol; ↑ GH
Tachycardia	↑ Catecholamines; ↑ FT_4; ↑ GH; ↑ aldosterone; ↑ cortisol; ↓ PTH
Body temperature	↑ Cortisol; ↑ FT_4 (heat intolerance); ↓ FT_4, ↑ rT_3 (cold intolerance)
Hypotension	↓ ACTH/cortisol; ↑ catecholamines (orthostatic); ↓ aldosterone
ECG changes	↑/↓ PTH; ↑ catecholamines (dysrhythmias); ↑/↓ ACTH/cortisol
GASTROINTESTINAL DISTURBANCES	
Nausea/vomiting	↑ PTH; ↓ ACTH/cortisol; ↓ insulin; ↑ catecholamines
Constipation	↑ Catecholamines; ↑ GH; ↓ ADH; ↑ PTH
Anorexia	↓ ACTH/cortisol; ↑ PTH
Diarrhea	↓ ACTH/cortisol; ↓ insulin (gastroparesis)
Abdominal pain	↓ ACTH/cortisol; ↑ PTH; ↑ thyroid
Polyphagia	↓ Insulin
Polydipsia	↓ Insulin
Weight loss	↑ Catecholamines; ↑ FT_4; ↓ ACTH/cortisol; ↓ insulin; ↓ AVP (diabetes insipidus)
Weight gain	↑ ACTH/cortisol; ↑ aldosterone (fluid retention); ↓ insulin (↑ glucose); ↑ ADH (fluid retention); ↓ FT_4, ↑ rT_3

FLUID/ELECTROLYTE IMBALANCES

↑/↓ ACTH/cortisol; ↑/↓ ADH; ↑/↓ aldosterone; ↑/↓ PTH; ↑/↓ insulin

GENITOURINARY DISTURBANCES

Polyuria — ↓ Insulin; ↑ PTH; ↓ ADH (diabetes insipidus)

Kidney stones — ↑ PTH (↑ calcium); ↑ GH

WEAKNESS/FATIGUE

↑ Catecholamines; ↓ FT_4, ↑ rT_3; ↑/↓ PTH; ↓ insulin; ↑/↓ aldosterone; ↑/↓ GH; ↑/↓ ACTH/cortisol

INFECTION

↓ Insulin; ↑/↓ ACTH/cortisol; ↑ GH

MOBILITY

↑/↓ ACTH/cortisol; ↑ GH

Tetany — ↓ PTH (severe)

PAIN/DISCOMFORT

↑/↓ ACTH/cortisol; ↑ GH

Bone — ↑ PTH; ↑ cortisol (fractures due to wasting of bone matrix); ↑ TSH, ↓ FT_4

Joint — ↑ GH; ↓ FT_4, ↑ rT_3

Headache — ↑ Catecholamines (pheochromocytoma); ↑/↓ ACTH/cortisol; ↑ GH; ↑ ADH

Neuropathy — ↓ Insulin

Parathesia — ↓ PTH (low calcium)

VISUAL

Visual field defects — ↓ Insulin (retinopathy); ↑ ACTH/cortisol; ↑ FT_4

Exophthalmos — ↑ FT_4 (Graves' disease)

(continued)

Hormonal Activity Suggested by Clinical Findings (continued)

CLINICAL FINDINGS	HORMONAL INFLUENCE
BEHAVIORAL/COGNITIVE	
Lethargy	↑ PTH; ↓ thyroid; ↓ insulin; ↓ ACTH/cortisol
Anxiety/nervousness	↑ Catecholamines; ↓ PTH; ↑ ACTH/cortisol
Confusion	↓ FT_4, ↑ rT_3 (thyrotoxicosis); ↑ insulin (hypoglycemia); ↑ PTH
BODY IMAGE DISTURBANCES	
Thick, oily skin	↑ ACTH/cortisol
Dry skin	↑ GH
Hirsutism	↓ FT_4, ↑ rT_3; ↓ insulin; ↑ GH; ↓ ACTH/cortisol
Diaphoresis	↑ ACTH/cortisol; ↑ androgens
	↑ Catecholamines (profuse in pheochromocytoma); ↑ insulin (hypoglycemia); ↓ PTH; ↑ ACTH/cortisol
Hyperpigmentation	↓ ACTH/cortisol (pituitary stimulated to produce ACTH and MSH)
Goiter	↓ FT_4, ↑ rT_3
Fat distribution	↑ ACTH/cortisol
Striae	↑ ACTH/cortisol

ACTH, adrenocorticotropic hormone; ADH, antidiuretic hormone; FT_4, free thyroxine; GH, growth hormone; MSH, melanocyte-stimulating hormone; PTH, parathyroid hormone; rT_3, reverse triiodothyronine.

22

Endocrine Laboratory and Diagnostic Tests

Conditions Resulting from Alterations in Endocrine Hormones

HORMONES	TARGET TISSUE	HORMONE LEVEL	EFFECTS	CONDITION
HYPOTHALAMIC AND PITUITARY HORMONES				
Antidiuretic hormone	Kidney	Increased	Water retention	SIADH
		Decreased	Water excretion	Diabetes insipidus
Thyrotropin-releasing factor	Thyroid	Increased	Impaired intracellular chemical reactions	Hyperthyroidism (Graves' disease, thyroid crisis)
		Decreased		Hypothyroidism (myxedema)
Adrenocorticotropin	Adrenal cortex	Increased	Metabolism, fluid, and electrolyte changes	Cushing's disease
		Decreased		Adrenal insufficiency (Addison's disease)

THYROID AND PARATHYROID HORMONES

Calcitonin	Bone	Increased	Changes in bone and calcium metabolism	Hypocalcemia
		Decreased		Hypercalcemia
Parathyroid hormone	Bone	Increased	Changes in bone and calcium metabolism	Hypercalcemia
		Decreased		Hypocalcemia

PANCREATIC HORMONE

Insulin	Muscle, body cells	Increased	Metabolism, fluid, and electrolyte changes	Hypoglycemia
		Decreased		Hyperglycemia (diabetic keto-acidosis, hyperglycemic hyper-osmolar nonketotic coma)

SIADH, syndrome of inappropriate antidiuretic hormone.

Comparison of Laboratory Findings in Diabetes Insipidus and Syndrome of Inappropriate Antidiuretic Hormone

LABORATORY TEST	DIABETES INSIPIDUS		SYNDROME OF INAPPROPRIATE ANTIDIURETIC HORMONE
	Central	**Nephrogenic**	
Serum			
ADH	Decreased	Normal or increased	Increased
Osmolality	Increased	Increased	Decreased
Electrolytes			
Na^+	Increased	Increased	Decreased
Cl^-	Increased	Increased	Decreased
Mg^+	Normal or increased	Normal or increased	Decreased
Urine			
Output	Increased	Increased	Decreased
Specific gravity	Decreased	Decreased	Increased
Osmolality	Decreased	Decreased	Increased
Water deprivation			
ADH stimulation test	Diagnostic	Diagnostic	
Water loading ADH suppression test			Diagnostic

ADH, antidiuretic hormone.

Comparison of Laboratory Findings in Hypothyroidism and Hyperthyroidism

LABORATORY TEST	HYPOTHYROIDISM	HYPERTHYROIDISM
Serum thyroid-stimulating hormone	>7 μU/mL	<0.1 μU/mL
Serum free thyroxine	<0.5 ng/dL	>4 ng/dL
Free thyroxine index	Low	High
Thyroid autoantibodies	Indicates autoimmune disease	
Thyroxine-binding globin	Used when free thyroxine is low but thyroid-stimulating hormone is normal	

23

Diabetic Ketoacidosis and Hyperglycemic Hyperosmolar Nonketotic Coma

Pathophysiologic Pathways for Diabetic Ketoacidosis (DKA) and Hyperglycemic Hyperosmolar Nonketotic Coma (HHNK)

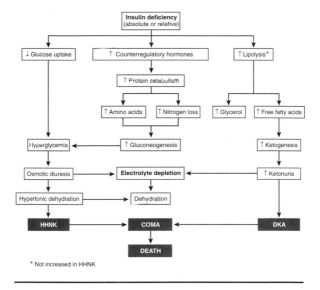

* Not increased in HHNK

Comparison of Features of Diabetic Ketoacidosis (DKA) and Hyperglycemic Hyperosmolar Nonketotic Coma (HHNK)

FEATURE	DKA	HHNK
Age of patient	Usually <40 years	Usually >60 years
Duration of symptoms	Usually <2 days	Usually >5 days
Glucose level	Usually <600 mg/dL	Usually >800 mg/dL
Sodium concentration	Likely normal or low	Likely normal or high
Potassium concentration	High, normal, or low	High, normal, or low
Bicarbonate concentration	Low	Normal
Ketone bodies	Present	Usually absent
pH	Low, <7.3	Normal

	Usually <350 mOsm/kg	Usually >350 mOsm/kg
Serum osmolality		
Cerebral edema	Often subclinical, occasionally clinical	Rarely occurs
Assessment		
Skin	Flushed; dry, warm	Pallor: moist, cool
Breath	Fruity, acetone	Normal
Vital signs	BP↓	BP↓
	Pulse↑	Pulse↑
	Kussmaul's breathing	Respirations normal
Gastrointestinal	Severe abdominal pain, nausea, vomiting	Mild abdominal pain, nausea, vomiting
Mental status	Lethargic	Lethargic
Level of consciousness	Decreasing	Decreasing
Urine output/fluid intake	↑Initially, ↓ with dehydration	↑Initially, ↓ with dehydration
Prognosis	8–14% mortality	10–20% mortality
Subsequent course	Insulin therapy required in nearly all cases	Insulin therapy not required in many cases

Example of Diabetes Management Protocols

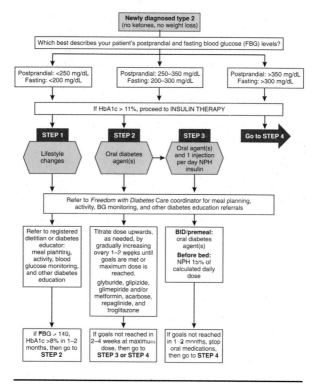

NPH, neutral protamine Hagedorn; R = regular insulin; UL = Ultralente. With permission from Via Christi Health System, Wichita, KS.

Example of Diabetes Management Protocols (continued)

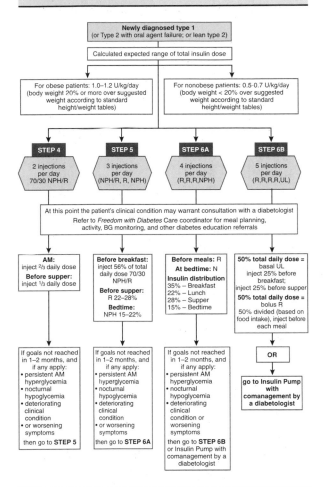

NPH, neutral protamine Hagedorn; R = regular insulin; UL = Ultralente. With permission from Via Christi Health System, Wichita, KS.

Complications of Diabetic Ketoacidosis and Hyperglycemic Hyperosmolar Nonketotic Coma

COMPLICATION	ETIOLOGY	TREATMENT
Cardiac dysrhythmias	Electrolyte abnormalities	Correct with alterations in IV fluids
Hyperkalemia	Acidosis, insulin deficiency, decreased renal tubular secretion, iatrogenic	Insulin/glucose, sodium bicarbonate
Hypokalemia	Potassium loss	Potassium chloride or phosphate added
Cerebral edema	Hyperosmolar consequences	Mannitol, intubation, ventilation
Pulmonary edema	Neurogenic, increased capillary permeability	Supplemental oxygen, diuresis
Hypoglycemia	Osmotic physiologic changes	Decrease insulin infusion, increase glucose infusion
Acute kidney failure	Severe volume depletion or papillary necrosis	Temporary dialysis

24

Diabetes Insipidus and Syndrome of Inappropriate Antidiuretic Hormone

Comparison of Diabetes Insipidus (DI) and Syndrome of Inappropriate Antidiuretic Hormone (SIADH)

	DI	SIADH
PATHOPHYSIOLOGY	Neurogenic: lack of ADH Nephrogenic, lack of kidney response to ADH	Oversecretion of ADH by tumor or overstimulation
ETIOLOGY	Neurogenic: idiopathic, brain injury, pituitary or hypothalamic surgery Nephrogenic: lithium, hypercalcemia, hypokalemia	Malignancies, especially lung, brain injury or surgery, pulmonary disease or mechanical ventilation, drugs
SIGNS AND SYMPTOMS	Polyuria, polydipsia, dehydration if free water not given Neurologic signs of hypernatremia related to brain cell dehydration	Weight gain without edema Neurologic signs of hyponatremia related to cerebral edema

LABORATORY DATA

Plasma osmolality	High, >295 mOsm/kg	Low, <280 mOsm/kg
Serum sodium	Normal or >145 mEq/L	Low, <135 mEq/L
Urine osmolality	Low, <250 mOsm/kg	Normal or high, >100 mOsm/kg
Urine sodium	Normal or low	>20 mmol/L
TREATMENT OBJECTIVES	Correction of underlying cause	Correction of underlying cause
	Free water replacement	Fluid restriction
	Neurogenic: ADH replacement	Hyponatremia: saline, hypertonic if symptomatic with
	Nephrogenic: thiazide diuretics	sodium less than 120 mEq/L

ADH, antidiuretic hormone.

Triphasic Pattern of Diabetes Insipidus (DI) and Syndrome of Inappropriate Antidiuretic Hormone (SIADH)

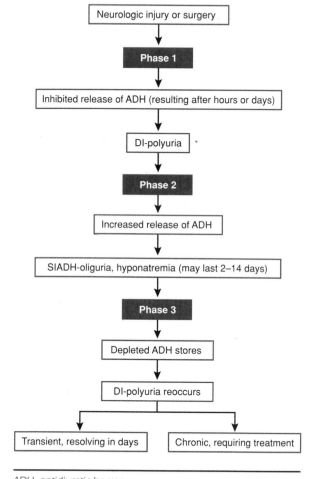

```
        Neurologic injury or surgery
                    │
                    ▼
                 Phase 1
                    │
                    ▼
   Inhibited release of ADH (resulting after hours or days)
                    │
                    ▼
                DI-polyuria
                    │
                    ▼
                 Phase 2
                    │
                    ▼
           Increased release of ADH
                    │
                    ▼
   SIADH-oliguria, hyponatremia (may last 2–14 days)
                    │
                    ▼
                 Phase 3
                    │
                    ▼
            Depleted ADH stores
                    │
                    ▼
            DI-polyuria reoccurs
                    │
          ┌─────────┴─────────┐
          ▼                   ▼
  Transient, resolving   Chronic, requiring
      in days                treatment
```

ADH, antidiuretic hormone.

Pharmacologic Therapy for Diabetes Insipidus

DRUG	INDICATION	ROUTE OF ADMINISTRATION
Vasopressin (Pitressin)	Acute	Subcutaneous Intramuscular Intranasal
Desmopressin acetate (DDAVP)	Acute/chronic	Intravenous Subcutaneous Intranasal
Lypressin	Acute/chronic	Intranasal

25

Thyroid Crisis and Myxedema Coma

A Comparison of Thyroid Crisis (Storm) and Myxedema Coma (State)

A Comparison of Thyroid Crisis (Storm) and Myxedema Coma (State)

THYROID CRISIS	MYXEDEMA COMA

PATHOPHYSIOLOGY

Excessive circulating thyroid hormone	Inadequate circulating thyroid hormone
Precipitating event: trauma, surgery, infection, emotional stress, medication overdose	Precipitating event: infection, trauma, emotional stress, exposure to cold, interruption of medications

PHYSICAL ASSESSMENT FINDINGS

Cardiovascular: tachycardia, atrial ventricular dysrhythmias, systolic hypertension	Cardiovascular: bradycardia, pericardial effusion, hypotension
Nutrition: weight loss	Nutrition: weight gain
Respiratory: dyspnea, tachypnea	Respiratory: hypoventilation, respiratory failure
Thermoregulation: fever	Thermoregulation: hypothermia
Neuromuscular: agitation, restlessness, emotional lability, wakefulness	Neuromuscular: decreased level of consciousness, psychosis, coma
Gastrointestinal: nausea, vomiting, diarrhea	Gastrointestinal: ileus

LABORATORY FINDINGS

Elevated T_4, free T_4, and FTI	Decreased T_4, free T_4, and FTI
Decreased TSH	Elevated TSH
Hypernatremia; hypercalcemia; elevated transaminases, creatine kinase, and alkaline phosphatase hyperglycemia	Hypokalemia, elevated cholesterol and triglycerides hypoglycemia

TREATMENT STRATEGIES

Medications: drugs that block synthesis (e.g., PTU), release (e.g., iodides) and/or cause peripheral conversion (e.g., glucocorticoids) of thyroid hormone; beta blockers; antibiotics (if infection present); antipyretics	Medications: thyroid hormone replacement (e.g., L-T_4), glucocorticoids, antibiotics (if infection present)

(continued)

A Comparison of Thyroid Crisis (Storm) and Myxedema Coma (State) (continued)

THYROID CRISIS	MYXEDEMA COMA
TREATMENT STRATEGIES	
T_4 removal: plasmapheresis, dialysis; ablative therapies (e.g., surgery)	
Supplemental oxygen as needed	Ventilatory support as needed
IV glucose and vitamins	Fluid replacement to maintain blood volume
Active cooling: blankets (taper once patient's temperature = 38°C), ice packs, fans	Passive rewarming
Identification and treatment of precipitating event	Identification and treatment of precipitating event

FTI, free thyroxine index; PTU, propylthiouracil; T_4, thyroxine; TSH, thyroid-stimulating hormone.

26

Adrenal Crisis (Addison's Disease)

Structures and Functions
 of the Adrenal Gland

Laboratory and Diagnostic Findings
 in Adrenal Insufficiency

Structures and Functions of the Adrenal Gland

STRUCTURE	HORMONE	FUNCTION
Adrenal cortex	Corticosteroids	
	Mineralocorticoids (aldosterone)	Cause the reabsorption of sodium and the elimination of potassium
	Glucocorticoids (cortisol)	Responsible for the metabolism of carbohydrates, proteins, and fats. Assists in the stress and the anti-inflammatory responses
	Sex hormones (androgens)	Thought to be partly responsible for the preadolescent growth spurt
Adrenal medulla	Catecholamines	
	Epinephrine	Causes actions similar to the stimulation of the sympathetic nervous system: vasoconstriction, cardiac stimulation, and bronchiole relaxation. Participates in the "flight or fight" syndrome
	Norepinephrine	Increases peripheral resistance (vasoconstriction)

Laboratory and Diagnostic Findings in Adrenal Insufficiency

DEFINITIVE LABORATORY FINDINGS	SUGGESTIVE LABORATORY FINDINGS
PRIMARY ADRENAL INSUFFICIENCY	**PRIMARY OR SECONDARY ADRENAL INSUFFICIENCY**
Increased serum ACTH	Hypoglycemia
Decreased urine ACTH	Hyponatremia
Decreased serum cortisol	Hyperkalemia
Abnormal ACTH stimulation test	Hypercalcemia
	Decreased serum osmolality
SECONDARY ADRENAL INSUFFICIENCY	Increased blood urea nitrogen/creatinine
Decreased or normal serum ACTH	
Decreased urine ACTH	
Decreased serum cortisol	
Normal ACTH stimulation test	
Abnormal metyrapone stimulation test	

ACTH, adrenocorticotropic hormone.

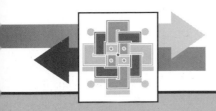

Gastrointestinal Disorders

27

Gastrointestinal Anatomy and Physiology

The Gastrointestinal Tract

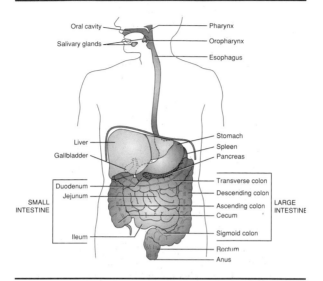

From Black JM, Matassarin-Jacobs E: Medical-Surgical Nursing: Clinical Management for Continuity of Care, 5th ed. Philadelphia, W. B. Saunders Co., 1997.

Cross Section of the Gut Wall

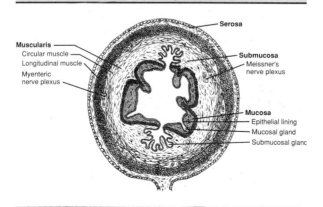

From Guyton AC, Hall JE: Textbook of Medical Physiology, 9th ed. Philadelphia, W. B. Saunders Co., 1996.

Swallowing Mechanism and the Structures Involved

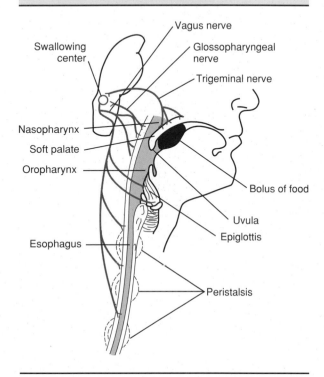

From Guyton AC, Hall JE: Human Physiology and Mechanisms of Disease, 6th ed. Philadelphia, W. B. Saunders Co., 1997.

Anatomy of the Stomach

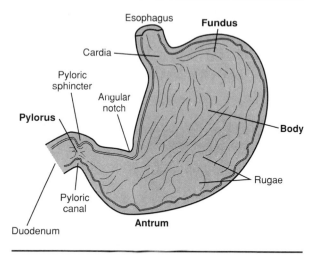

From Guyton AC, Hall JE: Human Physiology and Mechanisms of Disease, 6th ed. Philadelphia, W. B. Saunders Co., 1997.

Cross Section of the Small Intestine Wall

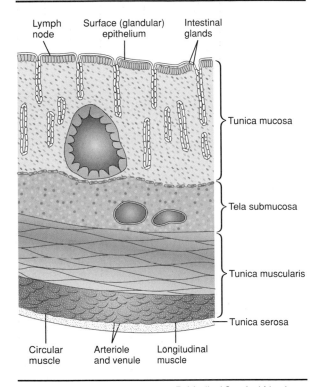

Lymph node · Surface (glandular) epithelium · Intestinal glands

Tunica mucosa

Tela submucosa

Tunica muscularis

Tunica serosa

Circular muscle · Arteriole and venule · Longitudinal muscle

From Black JM, Matassarin-Jacobs E: Medical-Surgical Nursing: Clinical Management for Continuity of Care, 5th ed. Philadelphia, W. B. Saunders Co., 1997.

Major Functions of the Liver

Bile formation
Metabolism of drugs and hormones
Substrate metabolism
Protein synthesis, including those associated with
    coagulation
Detoxification of noxious substances
Phagocytosis via Kupffer cells

Gallbladder and Pancreas With Connections to the Liver and Duodenum

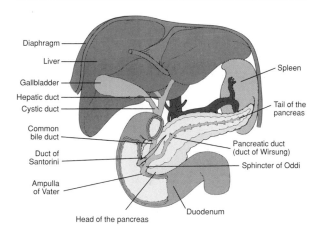

From Ignatavicius DD, Workman ML, Mishler MA: Medical-Surgical Nursing: A Nursing Process Approach, 3rd ed. Philadelphia, W. B. Saunders Co., 1999 (in press).

Splanchnic Circulation

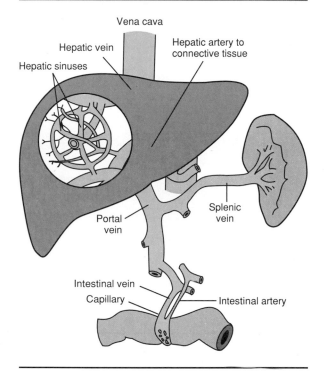

From Guyton AC, Hall JE: Human Physiology and Mechanisms of Disease, 6th ed. Philadelphia, W. B. Saunders Co., 1997.

Hormones of Digestion

HORMONE	ORIGIN	ACTIONS
Gastrin	Antrum of stomach in response to acetyl-choline stimulation of antral cells	• Stimulates secretion of hydrochloric acid by the parietal cells • Stimulates secretion of pepsin by the chief cells • Promotes stomach emptying • Stimulates pancreatic secretion (acinar cells)
Secretion	Duodenal and jejunal secretion in response to acidic gastric juice emptied from the stomach to the pylorus	• Augments the action of cholecystokinin • Stimulates pancreatic and hepatic bicarbonate and water secretion • Mild inhibition of gastrointestinal motility to facilitate digestion
Cholecystokinin (CCK)	Jejunal secretion in response to fatty substances in the intestinal contents	• Increases contractility of the gallbladder • Moderates inhibition of the stomach • Stimulates pancreatic enzyme secretion (amylase, lipase, trypsin)
Gastric inhibitory peptide (GIP)	Mucosal secretion of the small intestine in response to fat and carbohydrate in the chyme	• Decreases motor activity of the stomach • Slows gastric emptying • Stimulates secretion of insulin by the pancreas
Vasoactive intestinal peptide (VIP)	Small intestine secretion in response to the acidic gastric juice emptied into the duodenum	• Main effects are similar to secretion • Stimulates intestinal secretions to decrease the acidity of chyme • Inhibits gastric secretion

Adapted from Alspach J: Core Curriculum for Critical Care Nursing, 4th ed. Philadelphia, W. B. Saunders Co., 1991.

Neural Control of the Gut Wall

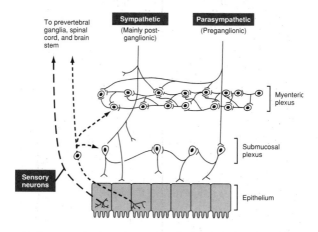

From Guyton AC, Hall JE: Human Physiology and Mechanisms of Disease, 6th ed. Philadelphia, W. B. Saunders Co., 1997.

Gastrointestinal Reflexes

REFLEX TYPE	NAME OF REFLEX	DESCRIPTION/EFFECT
Enteric nervous system based		Control: gastrointestinal secretion, peristalsis, mixing contractions, local inhibitory effects
Gut to prevertebral sympathetic ganglia and back to gastrointestinal tract	Gastrocolic reflex	Signals from stomach to cause evacuation of the colon
	Enterogastric reflex	Signals from the colon and small intestine to inhibit stomach motility and secretion
	Colonoileal reflex	Signals from the colon to inhibit ileal emptying
Gut to spinal cord or brain stem and back to gastrointestinal tract		Reflexes from stomach and duodenum to brain stem, back to stomach to control gastric motor and secretory activity
		Pain reflexes cause general inhibition of entire gastrointestinal tract
	Defecation reflex	Defecation signals travel to spinal cord and back to produce colonic, rectal, and abdominal contractions

Sites of Absorption

SITE	NUTRIENT ABSORBED
Small Intestine	
Duodenum	Iron
	Calcium
	Fat
	Sugars
	Amino acids
Jejunum	Sugars
	Amino acids
Ileum	Bile salts
	Vitamin B_{12}
Large intestine	Water
	Electrolytes

From Heitkemper M, Westfall U: Gastrointestinal Physiology. In Clochesy J, Breu C, Cardin S, Whittaker A, Rudy E, eds. Critical Care Nursing. Philadelphia, W. B. Saunders Co., 1993.

28

Gastrointestinal Assessment

313

Elements of the Gastrointestinal (GI) History

Personal Health History

Any preexisting GI condition
GI surgeries or injuries
  Oral, pharyngeal, esophagus, stomach, small
    bowel, colon, liver, gallbladder, pancreas
Abdominal surgeries or injuries
GI disorders or diseases, including peptic ulcer,
    polyps, gallstones
Past GI examinations (e.g., colonoscopy)
Prior gastrointestinal bleeding
Past hospitalizations
Blood transfusions
Major illness such as diabetes or cancer
Pancreatitis
Drugs: prescription; over the counter; recreational
Alcohol use, including type(s), quantity, patterns,
    consequences
Smoking or chewing tobacco
Recent travel history
Hepatitis or cirrhosis of the liver
Hepatitis vaccine

Family Medical History

Malabsorption syndrome
Familial Mediterranean fever (periodic peritonitis)
Gallbladder disease
Hirschsprung's disease, aganglionic megacolon
Polyposis
Colon cancer

Description of GI Symptom

Type
Onset
Location
Intensity
Duration
Frequency, if appropriate
Character, e.g., if pain—sharp, dull, burning; if
    diarrhea—watery, copious, explosive, undigested
    food
Aggravating and alleviating factors
Relationship to other symptoms, events, activities,
    e.g., food intake

Regional Elements: Mouth and Throat

Dental status
  Toothache or tooth abscess
  Pattern of dental care
  Dental appliances and fit
Gingiva
  Bleeding gums
  Sore gums
Mucous membranes
  Sores or lesions and location in mouth
Tongue
  Altered taste
Voice
  Hoarseness
  Changes in voice
Throat/swallowing
  Difficulty swallowing
  Sore throat

Regional Elements: Thorax and Abdomen

Heartburn
Dysphagia
Indigestion
Nausea
Eructations
Vomiting
  Character (color, consistency, quality, duration,
      frequency)
  Relationship to other symptoms/events/activities
  Medications
Hematemesis
Abdominal pain (characterize)
Jaundice
Dark urine
Fever/chills

Regional Elements: Lower Abdomen

Rectal condition
Hemorrhoids
Flatulence
Stools
  Patterns, aids
  Color, frequency, consistency, changes in stool
      shape, odor, gas, cathartics
Bowel regularity
Change in bowel habits
  Diarrhea
  Constipation
  Fecal impaction
Blood in stools

Oral Assessment Tool

CATEGORY	TOOLS FOR ASSESSMENT	METHODS OF MEASUREMENT	NUMERICAL AND DESCRIPTIVE RATINGS*		
			1	2	3
Voice	Auditory	Converse with patient	Normal	Deeper or raspy	Difficulty talking or painful
Swallow	Observation and tongue blade	Ask patient to swallow. To test gag reflex, gently place blade on back of tongue and depress	Normal swallow	Some pain on swallow	Unable to swallow
Lips	Visual/palpatory	Observe and feel tissue	Smooth, pink, and moist	Dry or cracked	Ulcerated or bleeding
Tongue	Visual/palpatory	Feel and observe appearance of tissue	Pink, moist, and papillae present	Coated or loss of papillae with a shiny appearance with or without redness	Blistered or cracked

Saliva	Tongue blade	Insert blade into mouth, touching the center of the tongue and the floor of the mouth	Watery	Thick or ropy	Absent
Mucous membranes	Visual	Observe appearance of tissue	Pink and moist	Reddened or coated (increased whiteness) without ulcerations	Ulcerations with or without bleeding
Gingiva	Tongue blade and visual	Gently press tissue with tip of blade	Pink and stippled and firm	Edematous with or without redness	Spontaneous bleeding or bleeding with pressure
Teeth or dentures (or denture-bearing area)	Visual	Observe appearance of teeth or denture-bearing area	Clean and no debris	Plaque or debris in localized areas (between teeth if present)	Plaque or debris generalized along gum line or denture-bearing area

*Values range from 8 to 24. The higher the value, the greater the risk of oral breakdown.

From June Eilers, RN, MSN, CS, University of Nebraska Medical Center, Omaha.

Abdominal Mapping Approaches and Underlying Organs

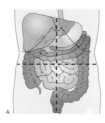

Right upper quadrant (RUQ)	Left upper quadrant (LUQ)
Liver and gallbladder	Left liver lobe
Pylorus	Stomach
Duodenum	Body of pancreas
Head of pancreas	Splenic flexure of colon
Hepatic flexure of colon	Portions of transverse and
Portions of ascending and	descending colon
transverse colon	Spleen
Kidney	Kidney
Adrenal gland	Adrenal gland

Right lower quadrant (RLQ)	Left lower quadrant (LLQ)
Cecum and appendix	Sigmoid colon
Portion of ascending colon	Portion of descending colon

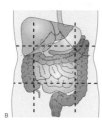

Right hypochondriac	Epigastric	Left hypochondriac
Right liver lobe	Pyloric end of stomach	Stomach
Gallbladder	Duodenum	Tail of pancreas
Upper pole of kidney	Pancreas	Splenic flexure of colon
	Portion of liver	Spleen
		Upper pole of kidney

Right lumbar	Umbilical	Left lumbar
Ascending colon	Omentum	Descending colon
Portion of duodenum	Mesentery	Tail of pancreas
and jejunum	Lower part of	Portions of jejunum and
Lower pole of kidney	duodenum	ileum
	Jejunum and ileum	Lower pole of kidney

Right inguinal	Suprapubic or hypogastric	Left inguinal
Cecum	Ileum	Sigmoid colon
Appendix	Bladder	
Lower end of ileum		

Elements of Adult Gastrointestinal Physical Examination

Oral and Oropharynx (Inspection and Palpation)

See Oral Assessment Tool, earlier
Gag reflex: present bilaterally

Abdomen (Gastrointestinal System Focus)

Sequence: inspection, auscultation, percussion, palpation

Approach: Four quadrants or nine sections (see Abdominal Mapping Approaches and Underlying Organs, earlier)

Inspection (Surface Characteristics Using Consistent Approach)

Skin color: moles; lesions, particularly nodules; scars—location, configuration, and relative size; spider angiomas
Contour: may need to measure circumference
Movement: respiration, peristalsis, pulsations
Symmetry

Venous return pattern
Hair distribution
Presence of tubes or openings, e.g., colostomy or
ileostomy; note locations, output consistency,
and pH

Auscultation

Bowel sounds using consistent approach (diaphragm
of stethoscope)
Frequency (normally 5-35/min)
Pitch (small bowel normally high pitch, colon
normally low pitch)
Character (clicks, gurgles, rumbling)
Vascular sounds (bell of stethoscope)
Location
Pitch
Timing (bruits over aortic, renal, and femoral
arteries; venous hums in epigastric area and
around umbilicus)
Friction rubs (diaphragm of stethoscope)
Pitch
Location
Relationship to respiration (normally not audible;
if present, often over liver or spleen)

Percussion

Presence of air, fluid, or solid masses using consistent
approach
Tones and tone changes
Location (normally tympany predominant sound
when there is air in stomach and intestine;
normally dullness over organs and solid
masses, including distended bladder)
Fluid wave of shifting dullness (may not be
detected if < 500 mL)
Liver border
Location: upper right quadrant and lower right
chest
Size: normal liver span ~6–12 cm (2½ to 4½ inches)
at midclavicular line

Palpation

Feel for areas of tenderness, muscle spasms, masses,
fluid with light palpation (~1 cm depth) using
consistent approach with pillow under knees if
possible: muscle resistance or guarding, rigidity,
tenderness, large masses (if detected, note surface
location)

(continued)

Elements of Adult Gastrointestinal Physical Examination (continued)

Palpation (continued)

Feel for organs in abdomen with deep palpation
(5–8 cm or 2–3 inches)
Liver edge: location, size, mobility, consistency, or
border smoothness
Gallbladder: normally not palpable below liver
margin
Masses: location, size, shape, tenderness,
consistency, mobility, surfaces, pulsation,
movement with respiration
Rebound tenderness: normally not present
(if present, note location)
Fluid wave: normally not present

Specific Abnormal Signs

See Abnormal Bowel Sounds, later

Rectal Area (Inspection and Palpation of Surface Characteristics)

Condition of anus and surrounding skin
Presence of hemorrhoids
Presence of tubes
Presence of large bowel contents (consistency,
quantity)
Palpable fecal mass above internal sphincter

Abnormal Abdominal Signs

SIGN	FEATURES	CONDITIONS
Blumberg	Rebound tenderness	Peritoneal irritation; inflamed or perforated appendix
Cullen	Periumbilical ecchymosis	Intra-abdominal bleeding; pancreatitis; ectopic pregnancy
Grey Turner	Flank ecchymosis	Intra-abdominal bleeding; pancreatitis
Iliopsoas muscle	Right lower quadrant pain when right leg elevated against tension	Inflamed or perforated appendix (inflamed iliopsoas muscle)
Murphy	Sharp pain; *abruptly* stops inspiration when palpating under liver border	Cholecystitis
Obturator muscle	Abdominal pain when right leg rotated at hip (internal and external)	Inflamed or perforated appendix

Normal Gastrointestinal Volumes, Contents, and pH Levels

LOCATION	DAILY VOLUME (ML)	CONTENTS	pH
Oral	1000–2000	Mucus, water, ions, H_2O, amylase, immunoglobulins	6.0–7.0
Esophagus	300–800	Mucus	
Stomach	1500–2000	Mucus, HCl, H_2O, ions, intrinsic factor, pepsinogen	1.0–3.5
Liver (bile)	500–1000	Bile salts, H_2O, ions, bilirubin	7.8
Pancreas	1000–1800	H_2O, ions, enzymes	8.0–8.3
Small intestine	1200–3000	H_2O, ions, mucus, enzymes, peptides	7.5–8.9
Colon	Variable	Mucus	7.5–8.0

Modified from Westfall U, Heitkemper M: Gastrointestinal physiology. In Clochesy J, Breu C, Cardin S, Whittaker A, Rudy E, eds. Critical Care Nursing, 2nd ed. Philadelphia, W.B. Saunders Co., 1996, p. 988.

Abnormal Bowel Sounds

STATE	BOWEL SOUND FREQUENCY
Diarrhea	Hyperactive
Early mechanical bowel obstruction	Hyperactive
Esophageal bleeding	Hyperactive
Gastroenteritis	Hyperactive
Hyperkalemia	Hyperactive
Resolving paralytic ileus	Hyperactive
Gastric bleeding	Hypoactive
Hypokalemia	Hypoactive
Inflammation	Hypoactive
Intra-abdominal bleeding	Hypoactive
Late bowel obstruction	Hypoactive (may be high-pitched tingling at obstruction)
Paralytic ileus	Hypoactive or absent
Peritonitis	Hypoactive or absent
Pneumonia	Hypoactive
Mechanical obstruction	Mixed hypoactive and hyperactive

Referred Pain Sites and Organs for Abdominal Contents

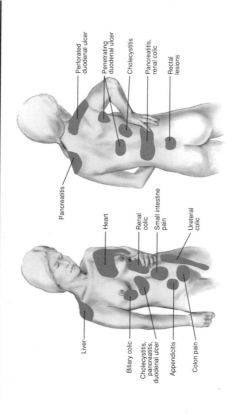

From Jarvis C: Physical Examination and Health Assessment, 2nd ed. Philadelphia, W. B. Saunders Co., 1996.

Gastrointestinal Variations Associated With Aging

Salivary flow	Decreased
Buccal mucosa	Less vascular and thinner
Tongue	More fissured
Gut motility	Decreased
Digestive enzyme secretion and protective mucus	Decreased
Intestinal bacterial flora	Bacteria available, participate less in digestion
Epithelial atrophy	Increased
Small intestine's ability to complete digestion and absorption	Diminished
Liver size	Begins to decrease at age 50 years
Cardiac output	Decreased
Hepatic blood flow	Decreased
Biliary lipids	May increase with age
Abdominal musculature	Thins
Pain	Less reliable symptom; intensity and quality may be diminished

29

Gastrointestinal Laboratory and Diagnostic Tests

Common Liver Enzyme Blood Tests and Normal Values

ENZYME (SERUM)	REFERENCE VALUES	COMMENTS
Alkaline phosphatase (ALP) and isoenzyme	*Norms:* Adult: 20–90 U/L at 30° C (SI units) 25–97 U/L at 37° C (SI units), 4–13 U/dL (King-Armstrong) ALP$_1$ 20–130 U/L	ALP is found mainly in bone and liver and also in intestine, kidney, and placenta. Since ALP is produced by several systems and cells in the body, its activity is classified as nonspecific; therefore, other liver function tests should be performed to confirm the diagnosis. In severe liver damage (i.e., cancer of liver, hepatocellular problems) serum ALP is greatly increased. ALP isoenzymes assist in identifying the origin of the problem. ALP$_1$ is of liver origin, and ALP$_2$ is of bone origin
5'Nucleotidase (5'NT or 5'N)	*Norms:* <17 U/L	5'NT is specific to liver cells. ALP and 5'NT are measured at the same time, since both enzymes are found in liver cells and are elevated in hepatocellular disease. However, serum ALP will be elevated in bone disease, but 5'NT will *not* be increased
Leucine aminopeptidase (LAP)	*Norms:* 8–22 mU/mL, 12–33 IU/L, 75–200 U/mL, 20–50 U/L at 37° C (SI units)	LAP enzyme is found mainly in liver tissue. Serum LAP is elevated in liver disease (i.e., cancer of the liver, viral hepatitis, acute necrosis of the liver, and extrahepatic biliary obstruction) LAP, 5'NT, and ALP tests are frequently ordered together to confirm liver disease. If only ALP is elevated and the other two enzymes are not, bone disease would be probable

(continued)

Common Liver Enzyme Blood Tests and Normal Values (continued)

ENZYME (SERUM)	REFERENCE VALUES	COMMENTS
Alanine aminotransferase (ALT or SGPT)	*Norms:* Adult: 5–35 U/mL (Frankel) 5–25 mU/mL (Wroblewski) 4–35 U/L at 37°C (SI units)	ALT/SGPT is found primarily in liver cells and is effective in diagnosing hepatocellular obstruction. AST/SGOT is found in liver cells; however, it is more specific to cardiac muscle and skeletal muscle. Serum ALT is slightly to moderately increased in cancer of the liver and cirrhosis. It is highly increased during viral hepatitis and drug hepatotoxicity
Lactic dehydrogenase (LD/LDH) Isoenzymes	*Norms:* Adult: 100–190 IU/L Isoenzyme LDH_5 6–16%	LDH is elevated in heart, lung, liver, and renal disease. To determine if the increased LDH is due to liver disease, LDH isoenzymes are measured. LDH_5 rises before jaundice occurs and falls before bilirubin level does
Gamma-glutamyl transferase/transpeptidase (GGT/GGTP)	*Norms:* Adult: Male: 4–23 IU/L Female: 3–13 IU/L Average: 0–45 U/L	GGT/GGTP is found mostly in the liver and kidney and small amounts in heart muscle, spleen, and prostate gland. It is a more sensitive indicator for liver disease than other liver enzymes (i.e., ALP and AST/SGOT). Elevated GGT/GGTP occurs in cirrhosis of the liver, alcoholism, cancer of the liver, viral hepatitis, and acute pancreatitis

From Kee J: Laboratory and Diagnostic Tests With Nursing Implications, 4th ed. Stamford, CT, Appleton & Lange, 1995.

Common Liver Function Laboratory Tests and Normal Values

LIVER FUNCTION TESTS (BLOOD OR URINE)	REFERENCE VALUES	COMMENTS
Bilirubin, total (blood) Indirect/unconjugated Direct/conjugated	Adult: 0.1–1.2 mg/dL 0.1–1.0 mg/dL 0.1–0.3 mg/dL	Serum sample Form bound to albumin Water soluble form
Urobilinogen (urine)	0–0.02 mg/dL	Conjugated form likely as unconjugated not water soluble
Proteins, total (blood) Albumin Globulin	Adult: 5.0–8.0 g/dL 3.5–5.0 g/dL 0.8–3.0 g/dL	Several proteins make up total value Electrophoresis enables amount and type of protein in sample to be identified
Prothombin time (blood) Factor II	Adult: 12–14 seconds 100% normal activity	Interinstitutional levels Variations Requires vitamin K
Fibrinogen (blood) Factor I	Adult: 200–400 mg/dL	Synthesized by liver Converted to fibrin by thrombin

(continued)

Common Liver Function Laboratory Tests and Normal Values (continued)

LIVER FUNCTION TESTS (BLOOD OR URINE)	REFERENCE VALUES	COMMENTS
Activated plasma (blood) thromboplastin time (APPT)	21–35 seconds	Screens for coagulation disorders; often used to monitor heparin therapy Prolonged in liver disease or vitamin K deficiency
Cholesterol (blood)	Adult: <200 mg/dL (questionable)	Synthesized cholesterol transported as low-density or high-density lipoproteins Liver esterifies ~70% circulating cholesterol
High-density lipo-proteins (HDL)	Male: 35–70 mg/dL Female: 35–85 mg/dL	HDLs carry excess cholesterol back to liver; high levels protective
Low-density lipo-proteins (LDL)	<130 mg/dL desirable >159 mg/dL high risk	Carry most of cholesterol from liver to tissues; high levels atherogenic
Very-low-density lipoproteins (VLDL)	25–50%	VLDL degradation is major source of LDL
Ammonia (blood)	Adult: 15–45 μg/dL 11–35 μmol/L (SI Units)	End product of protein metabolism; converted to urea in liver

Common Serum Proteins and Nutritional Status

SERUM PROTEIN*	HALF-LIFE	DEGREE OF REDUCTION		
		Mild	Moderate	Severe
Albumin (g/dL)	20 days	2.8–3.4	2.1–2.7	<2.1
Transferrin (mg/dL)	4–8 days	150–200	100–149	<100
Prealbumin (mg/dL)	2 days	10–15	5–9	<5

*dL = 100 mL.

Data from: Gibson R: Principles of Nutritional Assessment. New York, Oxford University Press, 1990.

Pancreatic Laboratory Tests and Normal Values

PANCREATIC TESTS (BLOOD OR URINE)	REFERENCE VALUES	COMMENTS
Amylase Blood Urine	Adult: 25–125 U/L 2-hr: 2–34 units 24-hr: 24–408 units	Interinstitutional variations Levels rise in acute pancreatitis, return to base in <5 days Levels low: pancreatic insufficiency Urine values 6–10 hr behind blood changes Refrigerate specimen
Lipase (blood)	Adult: 10–140 U/L	Pancreas major source In blood with organ damage Remains elevated after amylase returns to baseline

Test	Reference range	Notes
Fasting glucose (blood)	Adult 65–110 mg/dL	IV glucose may prevent "fasting" level Multiple ICU factors cause increase (e.g., physical stress) Multiple causes of decrease (e.g., liver damage, starvation)
Triglycerides (blood)	Male: 30–100 mg/dL Female: 35–110 mg/dL	Measures body's ability to metabolize fat Elevation with liver disease, alcohol use, pancreatitis, among other conditions
Serum calcium (blood) Total	Adult: 8.6–10.0 mg/dL 2.15–2.5 mmol/L	Circulating Ca^{++} ionized (50%); protein bound (50%) Hypoalbuminemia is common cause of low total calcium Cancer of liver, pancreas, and other organs shows high total calcium levels
Ionized	Adult: 4.65–5.28 mg/dL 1.16–1.32 mmol/L	Measurement may be used to track disorders, including cancer, acute pancreatitis

Diagnostic Tests for the Gastrointestinal System

TEST	DESCRIPTION/PURPOSE
Angiography	Radiographs of selected vascular beds and flow
Biopsy	Invasive procedure resulting in collection of tissue from organ or structure
Computed tomography (CT)	Radiographs producing cross-sectional images of underlying structures and tissues
Endoscopy (see Endoscopies of the Gastrointestinal System)	Uses fiberoptic instrument to visually inspect internal organs or tissues; may also be used for certain procedures or treatments
Fluoroscopy	Series of rapid radiographs that provide data about movement and location of organs within gastrointestinal tract
Magnetic resonance imaging (MRI, MR)	Uses magnetic energy sources that result in coronal, axial, or sagittal images without radiation
Nuclear scan	Visual inspection of organ or organ portion. Nonuniform radioactive uptake in tissues often indicates pathology; also used to detect motility within gastrointestinal tract
Radiography	Beam of short wavelength rays penetrates tissues; the amount of x-ray absorbed dependent on tissue density. Results transfer to photographic film Density can be altered with air or contrast media
Spiral computed tomography	Conventional computed tomography technique modification resulting in three-dimensional data composite
Ultrasound (sonogram)	Visual inspection of soft tissue structures through use of high-frequency sound waves

Diagnostic Tests and Nursing Actions for Gastrointestinal Disorders

DIAGNOSTIC TEST	INDICATIONS	CONTRAINDICATIONS	NURSING ACTIONS
Radiograph, abdominal Flat plate	Aid in diagnosis of intra-abdominal conditions (e.g., intestinal obstruction, organ rupture, masses, foreign bodies, abnormal fluid, or air)	Known early pregnancy	Protect gonads by shield
Radiograph, contrast Upper gastrointestinal tract	Visualize esophagus, stomach, duodenum, and into jejunum; pathologies (e.g., hiatal hernia, tumors, peptic ulcer, foreign bodies)	Allergy to contrast medium; inability to tolerate contrast medium or positions	Solicit allergy history for contrast medium; if needed, schedule other tests before barium use; pre- and post-test vital signs; assist with needed positions; check on limiting oral or enteral intake prior to test; actions to expel contrast medium; record stool color, amount, consistency

(continued)

Diagnostic Tests and Nursing Actions for Gastrointestinal Disorders (continued)

DIAGNOSTIC TEST	INDICATIONS	CONTRAINDICATIONS	NURSING ACTIONS
Small intestine	Visualize jejunum, ileum, cecum; possible pathologies (e.g., Meckel's diverticulum, tumors, Crohn's disease, visceral hernia)	Allergy to contrast medium; inability to tolerate contrast medium or positions	Solicit allergy history for contrast medium; if needed, schedule other test before barium use; pre- and post-test vital signs; assist with needed positions; check on limiting oral or enteral intake prior to test; actions to expel contrast medium; record stool color, amount, consistency
Colon (barium enema)	Visualize colon structure and filling pathologies (e.g., obstructions, fistulae, tumors, diverticulae, polyps, stenosis)	Allergy to contrast medium; inability to tolerate needed pre-test cleansing of bowel, contrast medium or positions	Solicit allergy history for contrast medium; if needed, schedule other test before barium use; pre- and post-test vital signs; assist with needed positions; check on colon preparation to use with patient; actions to expel contrast medium; record stool color, amount, consistency

Computed tomography scan	Visualize abdomen, retroperitoneal structures; tumors; cysts; abscess; fluid pocket, or air in cavity	Avoid barium if suspected perforation in gastrointestinal tract; allergy to contrast medium; claustrophobia; physiologically unstable	Solicit allergy history for possible contrast materials; if needed, schedule other tests before barium use; pre- and post-test vital signs; assist to lie still; give sedative; assess for allergic reaction, passing of contrast media
Ultrasound sonography	Characterize abdomen and retroperitoneal soft tissues; fluid pocket or air in cavity; abscess; can observe movement	Scar tissue over area to be studied distorts signal; dressings preclude access to skin above site of interest; fatty tissue can alter wave (obese patient may not be candidate); barium and air distort echo; open wounds limit lubricant use	Limit enteral or oral intake; inform patient of gel applied to skin over examination area; assist patient to lie quietly in supine/decubitus position; often some controlled breathing needed; pressure may be applied with transducer
Magnetic resonance imaging	Evaluate abdomen, retroperitoneal structures; abdominal neoplasms; abscesses, cysts; ascites, fluid pocket, or air in cavity	Internal metallic devices; attached external metal objects; claustrophobia; obesity; physiologically unstable; unable to maintain still position	Remove external metal objects, dental appliances; accurate history of internal metal/metallic implants; assist to lie still

(continued)

Diagnostic Tests and Nursing Actions for Gastrointestinal Disorders (continued)

DIAGNOSTIC TEST	INDICATIONS	CONTRAINDICATIONS	NURSING ACTIONS
Radionuclide	Visualize organs, elements of gastrointestinal motility; detect location of lower gastrointestinal bleeding	Pregnant or breast-feeding; some prostheses; hemodynamically unstable	Solicit allergy, pregnancy, nursing, recent nuclear exposure history; weight and age to use in calculating dose; note drainage tubes; remove metal; report if recently received barium, which may not have cleared tract. After test, monitor injection site; have visitors and pregnant staff avoid prolonged contact until nuclide cleared from patient's body

Peritoneal lavage	Abdominal blunt and penetrating trauma	Medical judgment about usefulness	Sterile catheter, equipment for insertion, sterile normal saline; observe insertion site for bleeding, leakage, infection; vital signs before and after procedure
Biopsy: organ specific, liver Percutaneous	Tissue needed for examination	Bleeding disorder; major ascites; infection at site	Baseline and follow-up vital signs; signed permit; ensure sterile procedure; turn to right side after biopsy; watch for pneumothorax, bleeding. Pain control measures
Liver (transvenous)		Bleeding disorder; biliary obstruction	Baseline and follow-up vital signs; signed permit; ensure sterile procedure

Endoscopies of the Gastrointestinal System

ENDOSCOPY TEST	INDICATIONS	CONTRAINDICATIONS	NURSING ACTIONS
Esophagogastro-duodenoscopy	Visualization of upper gastrointestinal mucosal structures for diagnostic or treatment plans; may locate source of upper gastrointestinal bleeding	Serious cardiovascular or respiratory compromise	Baseline and ongoing vital signs; safely administer IV sedation; ensure airway correctly placed; position to aid breathing; oral care before and after procedure; check for return of gag reflex; hold oral intake until gag reflex returned; side-lying position after test until alert; obtain signed permission form, sedation may be used
Colonoscopy	Visualization of large intestine structures for diagnostic or treatment plans; may locate source of lower gastrointestinal bleeding	Preparation exceeds patient's tolerance; perforating diseases of the colon; peritonitis; recent bowel surgery; serious cardiovascular or respiratory conditions	Baseline and ongoing vital signs; if on oral intake, clear liquids, then NPO; clarify bowel prep if needed; anticholinergics may be given; position Sims' or left lateral; check for clotting prior to test; often antibiotics before and after test for fragile patients; observe stools after test; may expel flatus; obtain signed permission form; sedation may be used

Test	Purpose	Contraindications	Nursing considerations
Proctoscopy/ sigmoidoscopy/ proctosigmoidoscopy	Visualization of sigmoid colon and rectum mucosal structures for diagnostic or treatment plans; may locate source of sigmoid or rectal bleeding		Baseline and ongoing vital signs; laxative or enema may be ordered before test; if acute symptoms, prep likely waived; obtain signed permission form
Endoscopic retrograde cholangiopancreatography (ERCP)	Evaluate biliary/pancreatic systems using contrast medium	Allergy to contrast substance; position contraindicated	Solicit history for contrast medium allergies and recent barium use; restrict intake prior to test; left lateral position; topic anesthetic into throat; mouthpiece in place; anticholinergics IV to relax duodenum and papilla; baseline vital signs and ongoing assessment; position to aid breathing; oral care before and after procedure; check for return of gag reflex; may experience abdominal discomfort, sore throat; after test, look for cholangitis or pancreatitis; obtain signed permission form; conscious sedation is used

Suggested Diagnostic Algorithm for Use With Blunt Abdominal Trauma

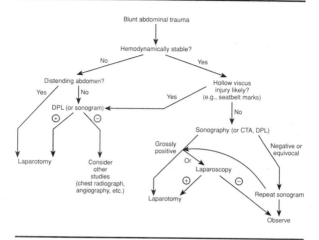

CTA, computed tomography of the abdomen; DPL, diagnostic peritoneal lavage. (From Elliot D, Militello P: Pitfalls in the diagnosis of abdominal trauma. In Maull K, Rodriguez A, Wiles C III (eds). Complications in Trauma and Critical Care. Philadelphia, W.B. Saunders Co., 1996, p. 146.)

Suggested Diagnostic Algorithm for Use With Penetrating Abdominal Trauma

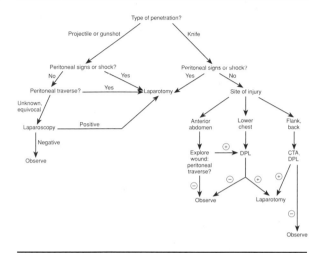

CTA, computed tomography of the abdomen; DPL, diagnostic peritoneal lavage. (From Elliot D, Militello P: Pitfalls in the diagnosis of abdominal trauma. In Maull K, Rodriguez A, Wiles C III (eds). Complications in trauma and Critical Care. Philadelphia, W.B. Saunders Co., 1996, p. 147.)

30

Acute Gastrointestinal Bleed

Diagnosis in Patients With Upper Gastrointestinal Hemorrhage

FINDING	OCCURRENCE*
Peptic ulcers	45%
Duodenal	23%
Gastric	22%
Gastric erosions	30%
Varices	15%
Esophagitis	13%
Mallory-Weiss tears	8%
Tumors	4%
Esophageal ulcers	2%
Angiodysplasia	0.5%
Other lesions	6%

*Total more than 100% because patients may have had more than one lesion.

Adapted from Silverstein FE, Gilbert DA, Tedesco FJ, et al: The National ASGE Survey on Upper Gastrointestinal Bleeding: I. Study Design and Baseline Data. Gastrointest Endosc 27:73–79, 1981.

Causes of Gastrointestinal Bleeding

Esophageal Bleeding

Esophagitis
Esophageal varices
Esophageal ulcers
Esophageal tumors
Mallory-Weiss tears

Gastric Bleeding

Peptic ulcer disease
Gastritis
Carcinoma
Angiodysplasia

Small Intestine

Angiodysplasia
Crohn's disease
Meckel's diverticulum

Lower Gastrointestinal Bleeding

Diverticulosis
Angiodysplasia

(continued)

Causes of Gastrointestinal Bleeding
(continued)

Internal hemorrhoids
Malignant tumors
Polyps
Ulcerative colitis
Crohn's disease
Rectal fissures

Causes of Esophagitis

COMMON CAUSES

Reflux esophagitis
Infectious esophagitis
  Candida esophagitis
  Herpetic esophagitis
  Cytomegalovirus
Acquired immunodeficiency syndrome
Caustic esophagitis
Radiation esophagitis
Medication-induced injury

RARE CAUSES

Crohn's disease
Ulcerative colitis
Graft-versus-host disease
Zollinger-Ellison syndrome
Thermal injury
Trauma

From Ott DJ: Radiology of the oropharynx and esophagus. In: Castell DO (ed): The Esophagus. Boston, Little, Brown, 1995, pp. 673–689.

Risk Factors Associated With Nonsteroidal Anti-Inflammatory Drug Usage

Prior history of peptic ulcer disease
Prior history of gastrointestinal bleeding
Age over 60 years
Use of higher doses
Concomitant use of corticosteroids
Tobacco use
Alcohol use

From Isenberg JI, McQuaid KR, Laine L, et al: Acid-peptic disorders. In: Yamada T, Alpers DH, et al (eds): Textbook of Gastroenterology. Philadelphia, JB Lippincott, 1995, pp. 1347–1430.

Diagnosis in Patients With Lower Gastrointestinal Bleeding

FINDING	OCCURRENCE
Diverticulosis	43%
Angiodysplasia	20%
Undetermined	12%
Neoplasia	9%
Colitis	9%
Radiation	6%
Ischemic	2%
Ulcerative	1%
Other	7%

Adapted from Boley SJ, DiBiase A, Brandt LJ, et al: Lower intestinal bleeding in the elderly. Am J Surg 137:57–64, 1979.

Assessment Findings in a Gastrointestinal (GI) Bleed

ASSESSMENT FINDING	SOURCE OF BLEEDING
Hematemesis	
Bright red blood	Upper GI
Coffee grounds material	Upper GI
Melena	Upper GI
Black, tarry, foul-smelling stool	rarely lower GI
Hematochezia	Lower GI
Bright red blood mixed with stool	rarely upper GI

Adapted from Elta GH: Approach to the patient with gross gastrointestinal bleeding. In: Yamada T, Alpers DH, et al (eds): Textbook of Gastroenterology. Philadelphia, JB Lippincott, 1995, pp 671–698.

Blood Products Used in Gastrointestinal Bleeds, Necessary Laboratory Tests, and Outcomes Expected

BLOOD PRODUCTS	TESTS	COMMENTS
Red blood cells	Crossmatch	Raises hematocrit 3 points per unit
Fresh frozen plasma	Blood type	In massive transfusions, may give 1 unit for every 5–6 units of packed red blood cells
Platelets	Blood type	6–8 units random = 1 unit single; goal is platelet count >50,000/mm^3
Cryoprecipitate	Blood type	Most commonly administered source of exogenous von Willebrand's factor (carrier protein for factor VIII)

Data from McGuirk TD, Coyle WJ: Upper gastrointestinal tract bleeding in emergency medicine, Part 1. Emerg Med Clin North Am. 14:523–543, 1994; Longstreth GF: Epidemiology of hospitalization for acute upper gastrointestinal hemorrhage: a population based study. Am J Gastroenterol 90:206–210, 1995.

Common Complications of Sclerotherapy

AREA AFFECTED	COMPLICATION
Esophageal	Ulcer formation Bleeding ulcers Perforation Strictures Dysphagia
Pulmonary and thoracic	Aspiration pneumonia Pleural effusions
Systemic	Low-grade fever Transient bacteremia

Adapted from Young HS, Matsui Suzanne M, Gregory PB: Endoscopic control of upper gastrointestinal variceal bleeding. In: Yamada T, Alpers DH, et al (eds): Textbook of Gastroenterology. Philadelphia, JB Lippincott, 1995, pp 2969–2991.

Histamine Receptor Antagonists

	CIMETIDINE	RANITIDINE	FAMOTIDINE	NIZATIDINE
Brand names	Tagamet	Zantac	Pepcid	Axid
Equivalent dosage	1600 mg	300 mg	40 mg	300 mg
IV infusion	Yes	Yes	Yes	No
Serum half-life	1.5–2.5 hr	2–3 hr	2.5–4 hr	1–2 hr

Data from Feldman M, Burton ME: Histamine$_2$-receptor antagonists. N Engl J Med 323:1749, 1990.

31

Hepatic Disorders

Clinical Findings of Liver Failure

BODY SYSTEM	PATHOPHYSIOLOGY	SIGNS/SYMPTOMS
General	Ineffective metabolism of carbohydrate, fat, protein	Decreased weight Muscle wasting Malnourished
	Inability to store vitamins and iron	Malaise, fatigue
Cardiovascular	Hyperkinetic circulation	Increased cardiac output, heart rate Systolic ejection murmur Bounding pulses
	Hypotension related to third spacing Fluid and electrolyte imbalances	Decreased blood pressure, renal blood flow Dysrhythmias Peripheral edema
Immune	Splenomegaly	Leukopenia Increased infection risk
	Decreased Kupffer cell function	Increased infection risk

(continued)

Clinical Findings of Liver Failure (continued)

BODY SYSTEM	PATHOPHYSIOLOGY	SIGNS/SYMPTOMS
Skin	Inability to conjugate bilirubin	Jaundice
	Inability to detoxify hormones	Palmar erythema
		Hair loss
	Elevated bile salts	Pruritus, dry skin
	Decreased synthesis of clotting factors	Bruising, purpura, ecchymosis
	Portal hypertension	Caput medusae
		Spider angiomas
	Hyperlipidemia	Xanthomas
Endocrine	Inability to detoxify or inactivate hormones	Peripheral edema
		Increased weight
		Moon facies, striae
		Testicular atrophy
		Gynecomastia
		Decreased libido
		Impotence
		Menstrual abnormalities
	Decreased glycogen related to decreased carbohydrate metabolism	Hypoglycemia

System		
Gastrointestinal	Elevated methylmercaptan levels	Fetor hepaticus, anorexia, nausea, vomiting
	Decreased fat metabolism	Steatorrhea, malnutrition, hyperlipidemia
	Portal hypertension	Hematemesis, melena, hematochezia
	Inability to conjugate bilirubin	Clay-colored stools
	Decreased synthesis of clotting factors	Epistaxis, gingival bleeding
		Heme + stools
Hematologic	Splenomegaly	Red blood cell destruction, anemia
	Inability to synthesize clotting factors	Nose bleeds, gum bleeds, disseminated intravascular coagulation, thrombocytopenia, ecchymosis
Neurologic	Inability to absorb fat-soluble vitamins	Sensory disturbances, peripheral degeneration, paresthesia, foot drop, nystagmus, ptosis
	Inability to conjugate ammonia	Personality changes, asterixis, change in level of consciousness
Renal	Decreased circulating volume	Decreased renal blood flow, glomerular filtration rate, urine output
		Elevated blood urea nitrogen, creatinine
	Inability to conjugate bilirubin	Dark, foamy urine (tea colored)
	Inability to detoxify hormones	Increased urine osmolality
Pulmonary	Ascites	Diaphragm elevation, shortness of breath, decreased lung expansion, pulmonary edema or effusion
	Increased 2,3-diphosphoglycerate levels	Decreased oxygen saturation and partial pressure of oxygen

Adapted from Covington H: Nursing care of patients with alcoholic liver disease. Crit Care Nurse 13:51, 1993; and Reishtein J: Liver failure: Case study of a complex problem. Crit Care Nurse 13:38, 1993.

Causes of Acute Hepatic Failure

Viral

Viral hepatitis, types A, B, C, D, and E
Acute alcoholic hepatitis

Viral Infections in the Immunosuppressed

Cytomegalovirus
Herpes simplex
Epstein-Barr
Yellow fever
Adenovirus
Varicella-zoster

Chemical

Hepatotoxic Drugs

Isoniazid (INH)
Rifampin
Chemotherapy
Acetaminophen (Tylenol)
Tetracycline
Valproate sodium (Depakene)
Phosphorus
Monoamine oxidase inhibitors
Alpha-methyldopa (Aldomet)
Nonsteroidal anti-inflammatory drugs (ibuprofen, Advil)
Drug overdose (acetaminophen)
Anesthetic agents (halothane)

Industrial Toxins

Carbon tetrachloride
Herbicides

Mushroom Poisoning

Amanita phalloides

Pregnancy

Fatty liver of pregnancy
Èclampsia

Medical Diseases

Wilson's disease
Budd-Chiari syndrome
Acute leukemia and lymphoreticular malignancies
Graft-versus-host disease
Reye's syndrome
Gram-negative septicemia
Ischemic/hypoxic injury/shock
Veno-occlusive disease after bone marrow transplant

Adapted from Smith S: Patients with hepatic disorders. In Clochesy J, Breu C, Cardin S, et al (eds). Critical Care Nursing. Philadelphia, W.B. Saunders Co., 1993; and Sussman N, Lake J: Treatment of hepatic failure—1996; current concepts and progress toward liver dialysis. Am J Kidney Dis 27(5):621, 1996.

Types of Viral Hepatitis

VIRUS	RISK FACTORS	RISK OF FAILURE	MODES OF TRANSMISSION	OTHER
Hepatitis A (HAV)	Poor personal hygiene Poor sanitation Household contact Sexual contact Employment or attendance at a day care center International travel	Low	Fecal–oral transmission via person-to-person contact Ingestion of contaminated food (e.g., raw shellfish or frozen foods) or water Parenteral transmission (rare)	Acute, not chronic Enterovirus Usually self-limiting Good prognosis Occurs in children > adults
Hepatitis B (HBV)	Homosexual contact Heterosexual contact Intravenous drug abuse Work in healthcare environment Transfusion of blood products Dialysis Tattooing or body piercing	High	Exposure to infected blood or other body fluids Perinatal transmission (rare)	Most common cause of fulminant hepatic failure Chronic carriers suffer no liver damage, but can transmit virus Can be asymptomatic DNA virus

	Forty percent of those infected have no known risk factors		
Hepatitis C (HCV)	Same as HBV	Moderate	Exposure to infected blood or other body fluids Fecal–oral transmission (rare) Perinatal transmission (rare)	RNA virus
Hepatitis D (HDV)	Same as HBV HBV infection	High	Exposure to infected blood or other body fluids Perinatal transmission (rare)	Seen with HBV as a co-infection
Hepatitis E (HEV)	Same as HAV (in endemic regions)	High, especially in pregnant women	Fecal–oral transmission Ingestion of contaminated drinking water	Enteric non-A, non-B Affects young and middle-aged adults Underdeveloped countries with contaminated water supplies Rare in United States

Types of Cirrhosis

TYPE	CAUSE	TREATMENT
Primary	Autoimmune bile duct destruction	Supportive and symptomatic
Secondary/ obstructive	Prolonged bile duct obstruction	Relieve the obstruction
Laennec's	Alcohol intake	Symptomatic and abstinence
Cardiac	Right-sided heart failure	Reverse heart failure
Postnecrotic	Liver cell necrosis secondary to infection, metabolism, toxicities	Symptomatic
Cryptogenic	Unknown	Symptomatic and transplant

Pathogenesis of Function and Renal Abnormalitites

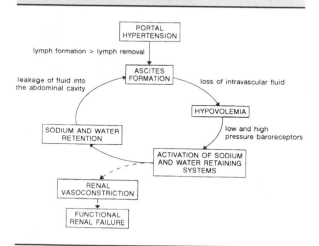

From Zakim D, Boyer T (eds): Hepatology: A Textbook of Liver Disease, 3rd ed. Philadelphia, W.B. Saunders, 1996.

Hepatorenal Syndrome: Clinical Presentation

Concentrated urine
Urinary sodium <10 mmol/L
Elevated blood urea nitrogen and serum creatinine
Oliguria
Hyponatremia often found
Urinalysis: mild proteinuria, granular casts,
    hematuria
Nausea and vomiting
Thirst

Encephalopathy Stages

STAGE	MENTAL STATE	NEUROMUSCULAR	EEG CHANGES
1	Subtle behavior and personality changes; irritable; mood swings; mild confusion; decreased attention span; slow mentation; slurred speech; uncooperative but rational; disordered sleep	Slight asterixis; normal tone/reflexes	None
2	Accentuation of stage 1; drowsy; inappropriate behavior; marked slowed mentation; confused and disoriented	Asterixis; reflexes brisk; increased muscle tone; impaired fine motor skills	Generalized slowing; abnormal
3	Sleeps most of time but arouseable; marked confusion; may be noisy or violent; incoherent speech	Asterixis; local/flexion response to pain; signature unrecognizable	Abnormal
4	May respond to pain only; coma possible	Asterixis absent; extends to pain; positive Babinski sign; hyperreactive reflexes	Abnormal

Prognosis for stages 1 and 2 is good. Stages 3 and 4 have a much worse prognosis. Once stage 3 to 4 develops, the patient is at risk for the development of multi-organ complications in addition to hepatic failure, and the mortality rate is high. Cerebral edema is estimated to occur in 75–80% of patients in stage 4 and is the leading cause of death.

Child's System of Liver Classification

PARAMETER	CLASS		
	A	**B**	**C**
Serum bilirubin (mg/dL)	<2.0	2–3	>3
Serum albumin (g/dL)	>3.5	3–3.5	<3.0
Ascites	Absent	Moderate	Tense
Encephalopathy	Absent	Grade I–II	Grade III–IV
Prothrombin time (sec > nl)	<4	4–6	>6
Operative mortality (%)	<1	10	>50

Types of Shunts Used to Treat Portal Hypertension

SHUNT	SELECTIVE	INDICATION	ANASTOMOSIS	OTHER
Portocaval	No	Most common	Portal vein to inferior vena cava	End to end or side to side
Splenorenal	Yes	Hypersplenism	Splenic vein to left renal vein	Decreased chance of variceal rebleed; shunt may thrombose
Mesocaval	Yes	Portal vein thrombosis; previous splenectomy; ascites	Superior mesenteric vein to inferior vena cava	Increased graft occlusion

32

Acute Pancreatitis

Pathophysiologic Progression of Pancreatitis

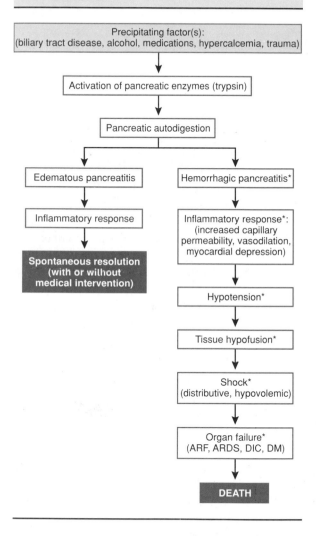

Precipitating factor(s):
(biliary tract disease, alcohol, medications, hypercalcemia, trauma)

↓

Activation of pancreatic enzymes (trypsin)

↓

Pancreatic autodigestion

Edematous pancreatitis

↓

Inflammatory response

↓

Spontaneous resolution (with or without medical intervention)

Hemorrhagic pancreatitis*

↓

Inflammatory response*:
(increased capillary permeability, vasodilation, myocardial depression)

↓

Hypotension*

↓

Tissue hypofusion*

↓

Shock*
(distributive, hypovolemic)

↓

Organ failure*
(ARF, ARDS, DIC, DM)

↓

DEATH

Causes of Pancreatitis

Biliary tract disease
Alcohol
Trauma
Hypertriglyceridemia
Hypercalcemia
Idiopathic
Infection
Shock
Medications
   Diuretics
   Steroids
   Transplant medications

Ranson's Severity Criteria

On Admission (or Diagnosis)

Age > 55 years
White blood cell count $> 16,000 / mm^3$
Blood glucose > 200 mg/dL
Serum lactate dehydrogenase > 350 IU/L
Aspartate transaminase (AST) > 250 Sigma-Frankel U%

During the Initial 48 Hr

Fall in hematocrit $> 10\%$
Blood urea nitrogen increase > 5 mg/dL
Partial pressure of arterial oxygen < 60 mm Hg
Base deficit > 4 mEq/L
Estimated fluid sequestration > 6 L
Serum calcium < 8 mg/dL

Hemodynamic Management of the Patient With Acute Pancreatitis

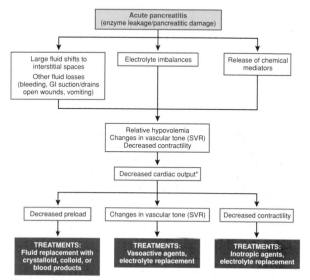

*Heart rate will change reflexively in response to the interventions used to optimize stroke volume

Factors Associated With Respiratory Failure in the Patient With Pancreatitis

Abdominal pain leading to guarding and decreased respiratory excursion

Pancreatic enzymes entering the pleural cavity either via the lymph circulation or through direct seepage and leading to pleural effusions

Increased serum levels of phospholipase A (an enzyme that catalyzes the breakdown of lecithin, a major component of surfactant), which decreases the amount of surfactant and leads to atelectasis and alveolar edema

Release of trypsin from the damaged pancreas causes widespread clotting abnormalities, particularly disseminated intravascular coagulation, which leads to microemboli in the lung and consequently causes ventilation/perfusion mismatches

Abdominal pressure from paralytic ileus or retro-peritoneal edema places pressure directly on the diaphram and compromises its ability to flatten during inspiration

Pulmonary hypertension secondary to pulmonary vasoconstriction

Complement-induced neutrophil aggregation, which increases capillary wall permeability and increases alveolar edema

Hypertriglyceridemia, which is often secondary to ethyl alcohol abuse, leads to the release of free fatty acids, which cause injury to lung tissues

Vigorous fluid resuscitation, although necessary, contributes to increases in lung water

Surgical Interventions for the Treatment of Pancreatic Pseudocyst

SURGICAL INTERVENTION	PSEUDOCYST CHARACTERISTICS	COMPLICATIONS
Excision	Small pseudocysts; easiest for pseudocysts located in the tail of the pancreas	Bleeding
External drainage	Used if fibrous lining of pseudocyst has not matured; used with infected pseudocysts	Fistula formation; skin excoriation; fluid and electrolyte imbalances; further infection; pseudocyst recurrence
Internal drainage	Mature pseudocyst; noninfected	Bleeding

Data from Butler RW, Smith SL: Acute Pancreatitis. Part II: Complications and Surgical Management. Aliso Viejo, CA, American Association of Critical Care Nurses, 1993.

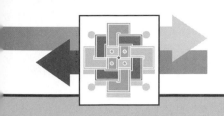

Neurologic
Disorders

33

Neurologic Anatomy and Physiology

Neurotransmitters and Their Actions

NEUROTRANSMITTER	ACTION
Acetylcholine	Excitatory
Dopamine	Inhibitory
Endorphin	Excitatory
Enkephalin	Excitatory
Gamma-aminobutyric acid	Inhibitory
Glutamate	Excitatory
Glycine	Inhibitory
Histamine	Excitatory/inhibitory
Norepinephrine	Excitatory
Serotonin	Inhibitory
Substance P	Excitatory

Neuroglial Cell Types

CELL TYPE	LOCATION	DESCRIPTION	SPECIAL FUNCTION
Astrocytes	CNS	Star-shaped; numerous radiating processes with bulbous ends for attachment	Bind blood vessels to nerves; regulate the composition of fluid around neurons
Ependymal cells	CNS (line the ventricles of the brain and central canal of spinal cord)	Columnar cells with cilia	Active role in formation and circulation of cerebrospinal fluid
Microglial cells	CNS	Small cells with long processes; modified macrophages	Protection; become mobile and phagocytic in response to inflammation
Oligodendrocytes	CNS	Small cells with few, but long, processes that wrap around axons	Form myelin sheaths around axons in the CNS
Schwann cells*	PNS	Flat cells with a long, flat process that wraps around an axon in the PNS	Form myelin sheaths around axons in PNS; active role in nerve fiber regeneration

*Some authorities do not consider these to be neuroglial cells because they are in the PNS.

CNS, central nervous system; PNS, peripheral nervous system.

Modified from Applegate EJ: The Anatomy and Physiology Learning System: Textbook. Philadelphia, WB Saunders Co, 1995.

Lobes and Functional Areas of the Cerebrum

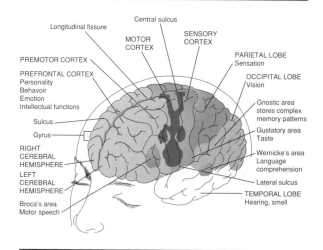

Redrawn and modified from Applegate EJ: The Anatomy and Physiology Learning System: Textbook. Philadelphia, WB Saunders Co., 1995, p. 167.

Cerebral Cortex: Structures, Functions, and Results of Injury

STRUCTURE	FUNCTION	INJURY MAY RESULT IN
FRONTAL LOBE		
Motor cortex	Voluntary motor activity	Weakness/paralysis on the side opposite to the injury
	Coordinates sequences of individual or combines muscle movements	
Premotor cortex	"Practice makes perfect" area	Difficulty with sequenced or skilled movements
Prefrontal cortex	Concentration, organization, and higher intellectual functions	Disorders of concentration, calculation, impulsivity, insight, and memory
Broca's speech area	Controls and coordinates larynx and mouth to produce words	Expressive or motor aphasia
PARIETAL LOBE	Receives and integrates sensations such as touch, pinprick, temperature, vibration, and proprioception	Sensory perception disorders

(continued)

Cerebral Cortex: Structures, Functions, and Results of Injury (continued)

STRUCTURE	FUNCTION	INJURY MAY RESULT IN
TEMPORAL LOBE		
Auditory area	Receives and integrates tone, loudness, spoken words, and music	Difficulty interpreting or understanding sound
Wernicke's area (usually left dominant)	Interprets all kinds of language (written, spoken, felt, or generated within the brain) Connects to Broca's area via the arcuate fasciculus	Receptive aphasia
OCCIPITAL LOBE	Receives and integrates visual stimuli	Visual disassociation/cortical blindness/field cuts
COMMISSURAL FIBERS		
Corpus callosum	Connects frontal, parietal, and occipital lobes	Impaired communication between the cerebral hemispheres
Anterior commissure	Connects the temporal lobes	

BASAL GANGLIA Caudate nucleus Globus pallidus Putamen	Exert coordinative effect on finer motor movements initiated in the frontal lobe, resulting in smooth, controlled muscle contraction	Discoordinate motor movements
RETICULAR FORMATION	Network of nerve cells modulating motor and sensory systems and influencing level of wakefulness	Loss of consciousness and coma
LIMBIC SYSTEM	Communicates with the hypothalamus, autonomic nervous system, and endocrine system to influence aspects of emotional behavior, particularly fear, anger, emotions associated with sexual behaviors, and also visceral responses to emotions	Disorders of emotional responses
Hippocampus	Recent memory	Disorders of recent memory

Diencephalon: Structures, Functions, and Results of Injury

STRUCTURE	FUNCTION	INJURY MAY RESULT IN
Thalamus	A major relay station of the brain. Processes all sensory and motor information. Coordinates and regulates all functional activity of the cerebral cortex	Loss of consciousness, loss of sensory function, and loss of motor function
Hypothalamus	Regulatory center for: Autonomic nervous system Body temperature Endocrine activities Thirst Satiety Emotional expressions Synthesizes "releasing" and "inhibiting" factors affecting the release of hormones from the pituitary. Synthesizes oxytocin and vasopressin, which are then stored in and released from the pituitary	Severe obesity or wasting, sexual disorders, hyperthermia, hypothermia diabetes insipidus, sleep disturbances, and emotional disorders

Brain Stem: Structures, Functions, and Results of Injury

STRUCTURE	FUNCTION	INJURY MAY RESULT IN
MIDBRAIN	Contains many connections to higher and lower centers of the brain. Involved with reflex movements of the head, eye, and neck in response to visual stimuli	A variety of motor and sensory disturbances, including paralysis, anesthesias, and cranial nerve deficits, particularly involving the eye
Cranial nerves	Cranial nerves III (oculomotor) and IV (trochlear) nuclei are located here	Cranial nerve dysfunction: extraocular movements and pupil constriction
Substantia nigra	Concerned with muscle tone	Discoordination (Parkinson's disease)
Cerebral aqueduct	Cerebrospinal fluid pathway	Hydrocephalus
PONS	Has many connections to the higher and lower centers of the nervous system and to the cerebellum	A variety of motor and sensory disturbances
Pnuemotaxic and apneustic centers	Controls rate and length of respiration	Respiratory failure
Cranial nerves	Houses nuclei for cranial nerves V (trigeminal), VI (abducens), VII (facial), and VIII (acoustic)	Cranial nerve dysfunction: motor and sensory to face, extraocular movements, and hearing
Cerebral aqueduct	Cerebrospinal fluid pathway	Hydrocephalus

(continued)

Brain Stem: Structures, Functions, and Results of Injury (continued)

STRUCTURE	FUNCTION	INJURY MAY RESULT IN
MEDULLA	Governs many basic functions of the body, including the rhythm of respiration, rate and strength of heartbeat, and cardiovascular tone. Mediates swallowing, coughing, vomiting, and sneezing reflexes	A variety of motor and sensory disturbances including paralysis, anesthesias, loss of consciousness, respiratory and cardiac decompensation
Pyramids	A bundle of fibers that are part of the voluntary motor or corticospinal tract. These tracts cross or decussate in the medulla	Paralysis
Fourth ventricle	Cerebrospinal fluid chamber	Hydrocephalus
Cranial nerves	Cranial nerves IX (glossopharyngeal), X (vagus), XI (accessory), and XII (hypoglossal) nuclei	Cranial nerve dysfunction: tongue, swallowing, and gag; neck weakness

Views of the Skull

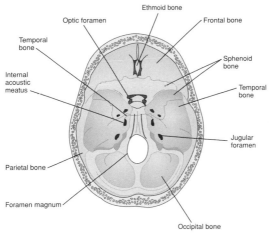

A

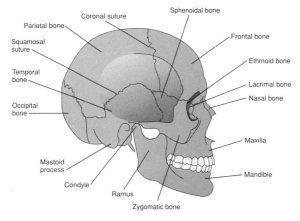

B

Ventricular System and CSF Flow

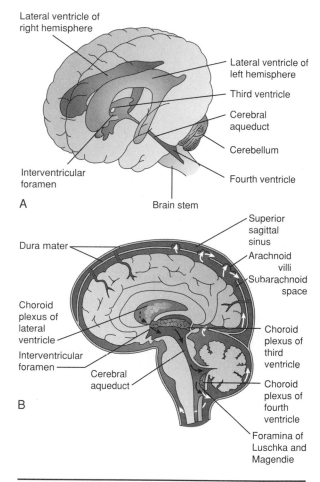

Lateral ventricle of right hemisphere

Lateral ventricle of left hemisphere

Third ventricle

Cerebral aqueduct

Cerebellum

Interventricular foramen

Fourth ventricle

A

Brain stem

Superior sagittal sinus

Arachnoid villi

Subarachnoid space

Dura mater

Choroid plexus of lateral ventricle

Interventricular foramen

Cerebral aqueduct

Choroid plexus of third ventricle

Choroid plexus of fourth ventricle

B

Foramina of Luschka and Magendie

Redrawn and modified from Applegate EJ: *The Anatomy and Physiology Learning System: Textbook.* Philadelphia, WB Saunders Co., 1995, p. 172.

Normal Components of Cerebrospinal Fluid

COMPONENTS	NORMAL VALUE
Color	Clear
Red blood cells	0
White blood cells	0–5/mm^3
Glucose	50–75 mg/100 mL
Protein	15–45 mg/100 mL
Chloride	700–750 mg/100 mL
Lactate	1.6 mg/100 mL

Cerebral Circulation

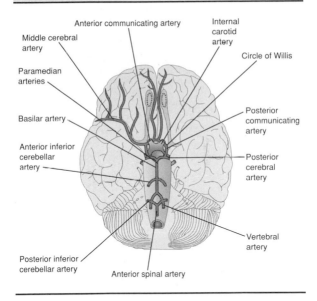

Areas of the Spinal Cord

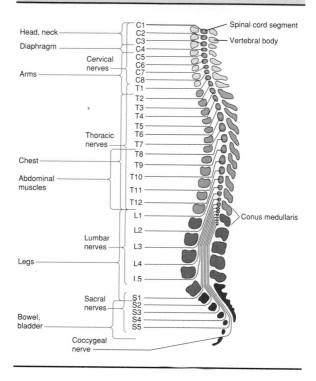

Twelve Cranial Nerves

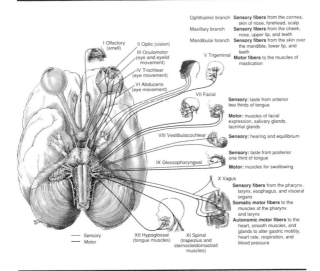

I Olfactory (smell)

II Optic (vision)

III Oculomotor (eye and eyelid movement)

IV Trochlear (eye movement)

VI Abducens (eye movement)

V Trigeminal

Ophthalmic branch **Sensory fibers** from the cornea, skin of nose, forehead, scalp

Maxillary branch **Sensory fibers** from the cheek, nose, upper lip, and teeth

Mandibular branch **Sensory fibers** from the skin over the mandible, lower lip, and teeth
Motor fibers to the muscles of mastication

VII Facial

Sensory: taste from anterior two thirds of tongue

Motor: muscles of facial expression, salivary glands, lacrimal glands

VIII Vestibulocochlear

Sensory: hearing and equilibrium

IX Glossopharyngeal

Sensory: taste from posterior one third of tongue

Motor: muscles for swallowing

X Vagus

Sensory fibers from the pharynx, larynx, esophagus, and visceral organs

Somatic motor fibers to the muscles of the pharynx and larynx

Autonomic motor fibers to the heart, smooth muscles, and glands to alter gastric motility, heart rate, respiration, and blood pressure

— Sensory
— Motor

XII Hypoglossal (tongue muscles)

XI Spinal (trapezius and sternocleidomastoid muscles)

From Polaski A, Tatro S: Luckmann's Core Principles and Practice of Medical–Surgical Nursing. Philadelphia, WB Saunders Co., 1996.

Spinal Nerve Plexuses and Involved Structures

PLEXUS	LOCATION	SPINAL NERVES INVOLVED	REGION SUPPLIED	MAJOR NERVES LEAVING PLEXUS
Cervical	Deep in the neck, under the sterno-cleidomastoid muscle	C1–C4	Skin and muscles of neck and shoulder; diaphragm	Phrenic
Brachial	Deep to the clavicle, between the neck and axilla	C5–C8, T1	Skin and muscles of upper extremity	Musculocutaneous Ulnar Median Radial Axillary
Lumbosacral	Lumbar region of the back	T12, L1–L5, S1–S4	Skin and muscles of lower abdominal wall, lower extremity, buttocks, external genitalia	Obturator Femoral Sciatic Pudendal

From Applegate EJ: The Anatomy and Physiology Learning System Textbook. Philadelphia, WB Saunders Co, 1995.

Sensory Pathways

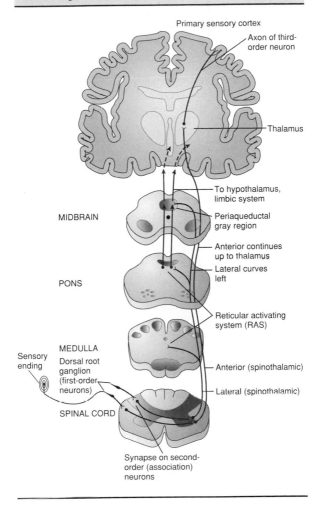

Primary sensory cortex

Axon of third-order neuron

Thalamus

MIDBRAIN

To hypothalamus, limbic system

Periaqueductal gray region

Anterior continues up to thalamus

Lateral curves left

PONS

Reticular activating system (RAS)

MEDULLA

Sensory ending

Dorsal root ganglion (first-order neurons)

Anterior (spinothalamic)

Lateral (spinothalamic)

SPINAL CORD

Synapse on second-order (association) neurons

Motor Pathways

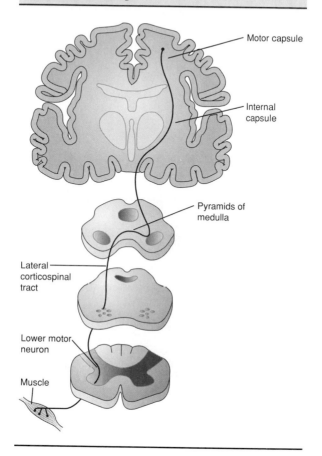

Motor capsule

Internal capsule

Pyramids of medulla

Lateral corticospinal tract

Lower motor neuron

Muscle

Sympathetic and Parasympathetic Pathways of the Autonomic Nervous System

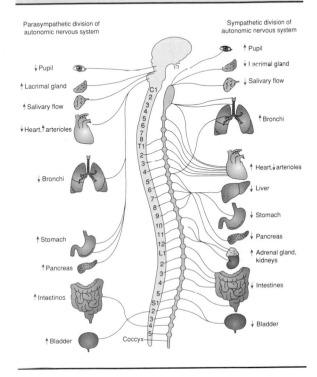

Parasympathetic division of autonomic nervous system

↓ Pupil

↑ Lacrimal gland

↑ Salivary flow

↓ Heart, ↑ arterioles

↓ Bronchi

↑ Stomach

↑ Pancreas

↑ Intestines

↑ Bladder

Sympathetic division of autonomic nervous system

↑ Pupil

↓ lacrimal gland

↓ Salivary flow

↑ Bronchi

↑ Heart, ↓ arterioles

↓ Liver

↓ Stomach

↓ Pancreas

↑ Adrenal gland, kidneys

↓ Intestines

↓ Bladder

Coccyx

Characteristics of the Sympathetic and Parasympathetic Divisions of the Autonomic Nervous System

AFFECTED STRUCTURE	PARASYMPATHETIC STIMULATION	SYMPATHETIC STIMULATION
Pupil	Constricts	Dilates
Heart rate	Decreases	Increases
Cardiac contractility	Decreases	Increases
Bronchi	Constricts	Dilates
Sweat glands	—	Increased secretion
Lacrimal glands	Increased secretion	Decreased secretion
Salivary glands	Increased secretion	Decreased secretion
Peripheral arteries	—	Vasoconstricts
Coronary arteries	Dilates	Constricts
Skeletal muscle	—	Constricts and dilates
Gastrointestinal motility	Increases	Decreases
Gastrointestinal sphincters	Relaxes	Contracts
Gallbladder	Relaxes	Contracts
Urinary bladder	Contracts	Relaxes
Adrenal medulla	—	Stimulates

Neurologic Changes Associated With Aging

AREA OF NERVOUS SYSTEM	CHANGES
Central nervous system	Cerebral atrophy Ventricular enlargement Localized neuronal death Axonal degeneration
Peripheral nervous system	Loss of myelinated fibers Slowed conduction of nerve impulses Vertebral degeneration

From Barker E: Anatomy and Physiology of the Nervous System. Neuroscience Nursing. St. Louis, C. V. Mosby, 1994.

34

Neurologic Assessment

Using the Acronym "OLD CART" to Explore the Chief Complaint

Onset: When did the symptom(s) first begin?

Location: Where do the symptoms occur? Have the patient point to or describe the anatomic boundaries or the location of the symptoms.

Duration: How long do the symptoms last? Minutes? Hours? Days? Weeks?

Characteristics: What do the symptoms feel like? May suggest that the patient rate any pain or discomfort on a rating scale of 1–10 with 1 = minimal pain/discomfort and 10 = the worst pain the patient can imagine. Is there a pattern to the symptoms? Do the symptoms move to other locations?

Associated symptoms: What, if anything, precedes, accompanies, or follows the onset of the symptoms?

Relieving and/or exacerbating factors: Can you describe those things that relieve the symptoms? What, if anything, makes the symptoms worse?

Treatments and effects: What treatments/remedies have been tried (especially any over-the-counter medications)? Which of these have worked, and how effective have they been?

Review of Systems for Neurologic Screening

AREA	SCREENING TOPICS
HEAD	Dizziness
	Headaches
	Pain
	Fainting
	Head injury
	History of stroke

(continued)

Review of Systems for Neurologic Screening (continued)

AREA	SCREENING TOPICS
EYES	Last vision check, use of eyeglasses or contact lenses Changes in vision (e.g., blurred or double vision, "floaters") History of glaucoma, cataracts, infections Pain Redness Discharge Excessive tearing Sensitivity to light Injury
EARS	Any hearing impairment, use of hearing aid Discharge, blood, fluid, pus Pain Ringing, any unusual sounds Infections
NOSE	Nosebleeds Infections, sinus infection Discharge Frequency of colds Nasal obstruction Injury Hay fever Changes in sense of smell
MOUTH AND THROAT	Changes in sense of taste Difficulty swallowing Last dental check, condition of teeth and gums Changes in voice, hoarseness Changes in speech, word finding, slurring Postnasal drip
MUSCULOSKELETAL	Weakness (paresis) Paralysis Muscle stiffness Limited range of motion Joint pain Arthritis Gout Back or neck problems Muscle cramps Deformities, congenital or acquired

Review of Systems for Neurologic Screening (continued)

AREA	SCREENING TOPICS
NEUROLOGIC	Fainting Dizziness Blackouts Loss of memory Loss of consciousness Speech disorders Disorientation Numbness Tingling Burning Stroke Tremors Unsteadiness of gait
PSYCHIATRIC	Psychiatric disorders (e.g., depression, suicidal ideation, mania) Mood swings Nervousness Hallucinations General behavioral change
SOCIAL	Drug and alcohol use Drug reactions or allergies

Mental Status Examination for the Conscious Patient

I. Level of consciousness: orientation to person, place, time, and events
II. Thought content
    A. Memory: **Short-term:** ask the patient to re-member 5–7 unrelated words (e.g., tunnel, basket, cat, hamburger, rain, tree, lamp) at the beginning of your evaluation. Test the patient's recall of this list later during the evaluation. Ask the patient to name the content of his or her most recent meal.
    B. Memory: **Long-term:** long-term memory can be evaluated by asking questions about the patient's date of birth and address.

(continued)

Mental Status Examination for the Conscious Patient (continued)

C. Judgment: Ask the patient what he or she would do if he or she found a checkbook with a name and address inside the front cover.

D. Calculations: have the patient count backward by 3s starting from 100.

E. Abstract thought: ask the patient what "a stitch in time saves nine" means.

F. Attention: Does the patient keep pace with the interview, or do you have to repeat questions or regain his or her attention?

G. Posture: is the patient sitting upright and midline; if not, what observations can you make about the patient's posture?

H. Affect: note and describe the patient's facial expression.

I. General information: give clues as to a current event and attempt to elicit the actual event from the patient (e.g., outcome of a recent election, an upcoming holiday).

Abnormal Pupillary Responses Due to Injury to Selected Cranial Structures

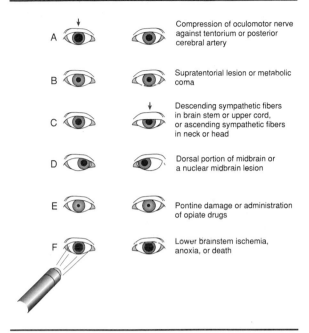

A   Compression of oculomotor nerve against tentorium or posterior cerebral artery

B   Supratentorial lesion or metabolic coma

C   Descending sympathetic fibers in brain stem or upper cord, or ascending sympathetic fibers in neck or head

D   Dorsal portion of midbrain or a nuclear midbrain lesion

E   Pontine damage or administration of opiate drugs

F   Lower brainstem ischemia, anoxia, or death

A, Ipsilateral pupil fixed and dilated; B, pupils small, equal, and reactive; C, unilateral Horner's syndrome (small pupil with partial ptosis); D, pupils midposition and nonreactive; E, pupils small and nonreactive (pinpoint); F, pupils fixed and dilated.

Extensive Evaluation of Muscle Function Testing

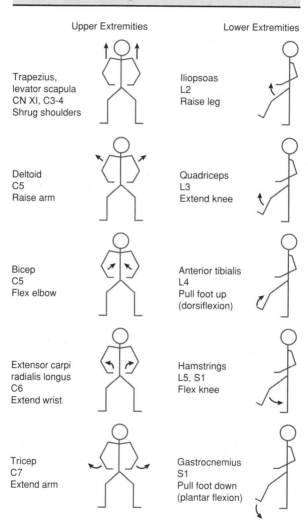

Upper Extremities   Lower Extremities

Trapezius, levator scapula CN XI, C3-4 Shrug shoulders

Iliopsoas L2 Raise leg

Deltoid C5 Raise arm

Quadriceps L3 Extend knee

Bicep C5 Flex elbow

Anterior tibialis L4 Pull foot up (dorsiflexion)

Extensor carpi radialis longus C6 Extend wrist

Hamstrings L5, S1 Flex knee

Tricep C7 Extend arm

Gastrocnemius S1 Pull foot down (plantar flexion)

Courtesy of Phyllis Dubendorf, Drexel Hill, PA.

Oculocephalic Reflex

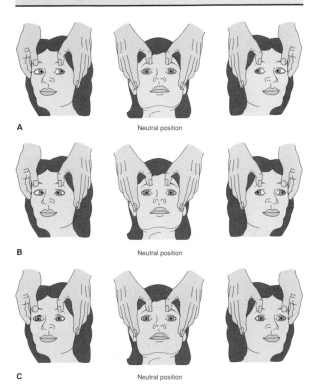

A, Normal response; B, abnormal response indicating some degree of brain stem injury; C, absent response.

Oculovestibular (Iced Water Caloric) Reflex

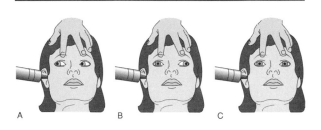

A, Normal response; B, abnormal response (disconjugate eye movement) indicating brain stem injury; C, absent response indicating significant brain stem injury.

Abnormal Respiratory Patterns Associated With Coma

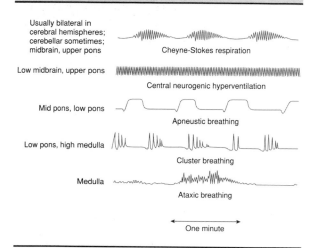

Usually bilateral in cerebral hemispheres; cerebellar sometimes; midbrain, upper pons
Cheyne-Stokes respiration

Low midbrain, upper pons
Central neurogenic hyperventilation

Mid pons, low pons
Apneustic breathing

Low pons, high medulla
Cluster breathing

Medulla
Ataxic breathing

←—— One minute ——→

Motor Strength Scoring

The following scale is often used as an objective measure of motor strength:

5: Normal strength, resists equally opposing force
4: Offers resistance but able to be overcome by examiner
3: Able to overcome gravity (e.g., moves in a vertical plane but no resistance to examiner)
2: Cannot oppose gravity, moves only in horizontal plane
1: Flicker of muscle movement, visible or palpable
0: *No* movement

Range of motion measures joint mobility, and some adaptation in technique may be required when assessing for muscle strength.

Deep Tendon Reflexes

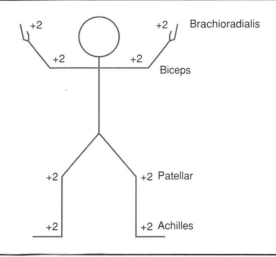

+2 Brachioradialis

+2 Biceps

+2 Patellar

+2 Achilles

Effects of Aging on the Nervous System

SYSTEM	EFFECTS OF AGING
GENERAL	Decreased brain size causing traction on bridging veins and increasing risk for subdural hemorrhage secondary to trauma
	Decreased number of functional neurons
	Decreased vibratory and position sense in lower extremities
	Decreased two-point discrimination
	Decreased reflexes and reaction times
	Increased sleep disturbances, decreasing REM and stage 4 sleep
	Degenerative connective tissue and bone may increase risk for spinal cord compression
	Significant risk for depression
	Increased risk for stroke, Parkinson's disease, and dementia

(continued)

Effects of Aging on the Nervous System (continued)

SYSTEM	EFFECTS OF AGING
VISION	Presbyopia (decreased near vision) Arcus senilis (opaque white ring around the periphery of the cornea) Development of cataracts Smaller, less reactive pupils Slower adaptation to darkness Decreased color discrimination (especially between blue and green) Decreased upward and downward gaze
HEARING	Presbycusis Deterioration of hair and bone Loss of "f," "s," "th," "ch," and "sh" sounds
TASTE	Decreased number of taste buds Xerostomia (decreased saliva production by one-third) Atrophy of the oral mucosa
MOTOR FUNCTION	Overall strength decreases by 10–45% due to loss of motor cortex and spinal cord tracts for motor function Decreased velocity of peripheral nerve conduction Loss of total number of muscle cells Decreased number and bulk of muscle fibers Stooped posture related to degeneration of intervertebral discs Short, shuffling gait with loss of arm swing on walking Decreased dorsiflexion of foot

35

Neurologic Laboratory and Diagnostic Tests

Computed Tomography (CT) Color of Various Substances

SUBSTANCE	COLOR ON SCAN
Bone	White
Blood	Off white
Tissue	Shaded gray
Cerebrospinal fluid	Off black
Air	Black

Electroencephalograph Wave Classification

WAVE	CYCLES PER SECOND	FINDINGS
Delta	1–4	Seen in sleep Not normal in awake adult
Theta	4–8	Originates from temporal and parietal lobes Normal in drowsiness
Alpha	8–13	Most prominent in occipital leads Considered normal in adult Can be blocked by beta waves
Beta	13–35	Most prominent in frontal and central areas Opening of eyes, mental activity, anxiety, or apprehension

Electroencephalograph Patterns

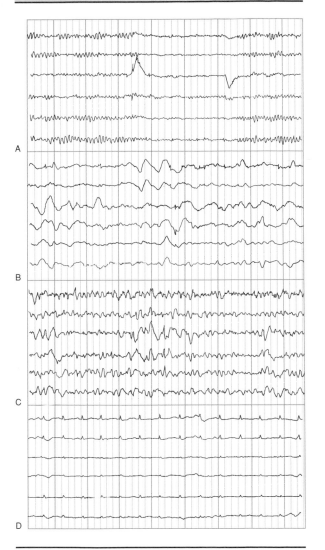

A, Normal EEG. *B*, Generalized slowing. *C*, Temporal spikes (seizures). *D*, Electrocerebral silence.

Transcranial Doppler Waveforms

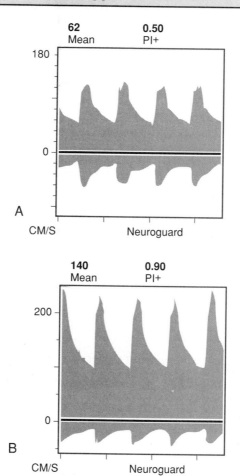

A, Normal. *B,* Cerebral vasospasm.

Comparison of Intracranial Pressure (ICP) Monitoring Devices

ICP MONITORING DEVICES	CATHETER PLACEMENT	ADVANTAGES	DISADVANTAGES
Intraventricular catheter	Anterior horn of the lateral ventricle	Drain CSF Most accurate and reliable for ICP	Most difficult to place Highest risk of infection Need for transducer leveling and repositioning with head movement Unable to obtain accurate ICP reading when draining CSF
Subarachnoid	Subarachnoid space	No penetration of the parenchyma, less risk of infection or hemorrhage Easier to place than intraventricular catheter Useful when unable to place intraventricular catheter due to edema	Accuracy and reliability over time are poor May be unable to drain CSF Can become clotted off with blood clot or brain tissue Requires intact skull for accurate ICP readings Need for transducer leveling and repositioning with head movement

(continued)

Comparison of Intracranial Pressure (ICP) Monitoring Devices (continued)

ICP MONITORING DEVICES	CATHETER PLACEMENT	ADVANTAGES	DISADVANTAGES
Epidural	Epidural space	No penetration of dura layer Easiest to place Low infection risk Can be used for longer periods of time No adjustment of transducer with head movement needed	Indirect measurement of ICP/questionable accuracy Unable to drain CSF Unable to recalibrate or rezero after placement
Fiberoptic	Epidural, subarachnoid, or parenchymal space	Accurate and reliable Easy to place Can be used longer term No adjustment of transducer with head movement needed	Unable to drain CSF Unable to recalibrate or rezero after placement Requires large investment in equipment/hardware for fiberoptics Fiberoptics can be broken if cable is kinked

CSF, cerebrospinal fluid.

Location of Intracranial Pressure Monitors

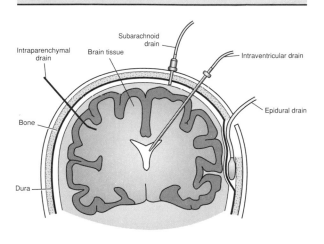

Normal Intracranial Pressure Waveform

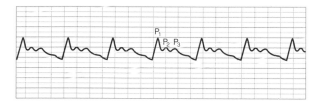

Increased Intracranial Pressure Waveform

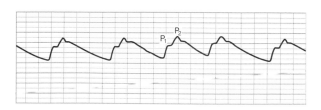

Note that P_2 is greater than P_1.

Nursing Considerations During Intracranial Pressure (ICP) Monitoring

NURSING CONSIDERATIONS	RATIONALE
Maintain knowledge of the indications for ICP monitoring	Timely assembling of equipment is required due to the critical condition of the patient
Assemble equipment accurately	Important to know the type of ICP monitor For accurate ICP readings: the intraventricular catheter needs to be leveled, with zero being the outer canthus of the eye or the foramen of Monro; a physician's order must be obtained for the level of the drainage system above that zero point For other ICP monitoring devices, the transducers may be at the level of the outer canthus of the eye and zeroed appropriately Fiberoptic monitors are calibrated prior to insertion, and level of the device is not a factor Use strict sterile technique when setting up the ICP monitor Do not connect the transducer of any ICP monitor to a flush system
Keep patient free from infection	Maintain aseptic technique with all dressing changes and trouble-shooting of devices Keep all stopcocks in closed position and sterile Monitor insertion site for redness, swelling, warmth, or drainage Administer antibiotics as prescribed

Nursing Considerations During Intracranial Pressure (ICP) Monitoring

NURSING CONSIDERATIONS	RATIONALE
Monitor vital signs and neurologic status frequently	Record ICP readings with the patient in the same position according to the physician's order or the nursing standards of care Record ICP readings more frequently if unstable Record high and mode ICP if the monitor is continuous Begin medical and nursing interventions as prescribed for ICP >20 mm Hg or CPP <60–70 mm Hg
Monitor the effect of nursing interventions on the patient's ICP	Space out nursing interventions: ICP has been shown to increase with turning of the patient and with endotracheal suctioning. Bathing may or may not increase ICP Noise has been associated with increases in ICP ICP should return to baseline in no more than 4–5 min after stimulation or a nursing care activity
Document thoroughly	Document: ICP/CPP values, waveforms, neurologic assessments, type of ICP monitoring device, location and condition of insertion site, dressing changes, amount and color of cerebrospinal drainage. This will provide the necessary information for evaluating patient trends and the effectiveness of medical and nursing therapies

(continued)

Nursing Considerations During Intracranial Pressure (ICP) Monitoring (continued)

NURSING CONSIDERATIONS	RATIONALE

Troubleshoot the ICP monitoring system as needed	For damped waveform:
	  Compare waveform with outgoing RN
	  Change scales on monitor if appropriate
	  Check all stopcocks/ connections
	  Check level of monitor if appropriate
	  Rezero monitor/transducer
	  Look for evidence of pulsatile fluid in catheter if appropriate
	  Try to drain system if physician's order in place
	  Manually flush transducer *only*
	  Call neurosurgery/ physician to flush monitoring system if appropriate
	For absent waveform:
	  Check all stopcocks/ connections
	  Check level of monitor if appropriate
	  Rezero monitor/transducer
	  Look for evidence of pulsatile fluid in catheter if appropriate
	  Try to drain system if physician's order in place
	  Manually flush transducer *only*
	  Call neurosurgeon/ physician to flush/ replace monitoring system

CPP, cerebral perfusion pressure.

Nursing Considerations for Transport of the Patient With a Neurologic Deficit

NURSING ACTIONS	RATIONALE
Confirm with precise time and location of test with department	Excessive waiting outside the intensive care unit can place the patient at risk for deterioration
Notify ancillary departments whose personnel will need to accompany patient Respiratory therapy, nursing Assistants/technicians	Give other personnel as much time as possible to prepare for patient's needs, such as gathering transport ventilator, pressure transducers, and pulse oximetry monitors
Gather transport supplies: Emergency medications/ pack Sedatives if needed Transport monitor Routine medications needed during lengthy procedure (diuretics, antihypertensives) Emergency intubation equipment	Ensure appropriate patient monitoring to maintain standards of care while at the test; emergency preparedness while off the unit in a remote location is required
Attach patient to transport monitor and transport ventilator/Ambu bag as required	Minimally, electrocardiogram, blood pressure, and pulse oximetry should be monitored. ICP monitoring is vital in the patient requiring ICP assessment or therapy
Ensure all equipment (e.g., IVs, monitors, blankets, beds, oxygen) are unplugged. Check the status of all equipment's battery power at this time	Ensures a smooth transport out of the room and enough battery power to provide uninterrupted delivery of therapy
Transport to the procedure department	If the patient is traveling with a ventilator and other equipment, ensure passageways and elevators are accessible to avoid delays

(continued)

Nursing Considerations for Transport of the Patient With a Neurologic Deficit (continued)

NURSING ACTIONS	RATIONALE
Assist with transferring patient to the diagnostic table	Three to four people will be needed to transfer the patient safely
Position monitoring equipment and other devices so that they can be observed easily during the test	Allows the nurse to assess the patient continually during the test
Perform neurologic and hemodynamic assessment prior to test	Establishes patient stability after transport and baseline data prior to the start of the test
Monitor and record patient parameters (electrocardiogram, blood pressure, pulse oximetry, and ICP) during examination	Provides documentation of the patient's physiologic responses during test
Transfer patient and equipment back to stretcher/bed and then transport patient to intensive care unit	Three to four people will be needed to transfer the patient safely and to transport the patient to the intensive care unit

36

Acute Head Injury

Symptoms Associated With a Mild Traumatic Brain Injury

Area	Symptoms
Somatic	Headache, dizziness, nausea and vomiting, blurred vision, tinnitus and hearing difficulties, drowsiness, seizures (rare)
Cognitive	Amnesia of event, impaired attention and concentration, impaired short-term memory, disorientation and confusion, slow thinking and information processing, poor judgment, mental fatigue
Emotional–behavioral	Agitation, irritability, apathy, depression, emotional instability, sleep disturbance, lower tolerance for frustration, loss of sexual drive, intolerance to ethyl alcohol

Systemic and Intracranial Events That Affect Perfusion

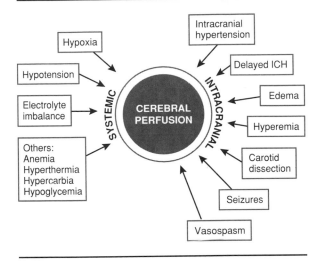

Mechanisms of Autoregulation

MECHANISM		VASOCONSTRICTION	VASODILATION
Metabolic	↑ Demand		X
	↓ Demand	X	
Myogenic	↑ SABP	X	
	↓ SABP		X
Chemical	↑ PaO_2, ↓ $PaCO_2$, ↑ pH	X	
	↓ PaO_2, ↑ $PaCO_2$, ↓ pH		X

$PaCO_2$, partial pressure of arterial carbon dioxide; PaO_2, partial pressure of arterial oxygen; SABP, systemic arterial blood pressure.

Ischemia Cascade

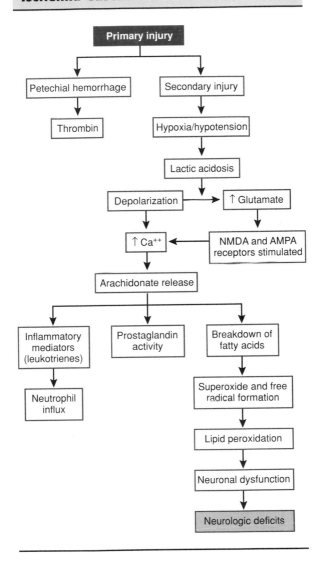

Glasgow Coma Scale

RESPONSE	RATING
EYE OPENING (1–4)	
Opens eyes spontaneously	4
Opens eyes to verbal	3
Opens eyes to pain	2
No eye opening	1
BEST VERBAL (1–5)	
Oriented	5
Confused (disoriented)	4
Inappropriate (swearing, yelling)	3
Incomprehensible sounds (moans)	2
None	1
Intubate	1T
MOTOR (6–1)	
Follows commands	6
Localizes to pain (purposeful)	5*
Normal flexion (withdrawal)	4*
Abnormal flexion (decortication)	3*
Extension (decerebration)	2*
None	1*

*Noxious stimuli are best applied using a central stimulus, to avoid eliciting a spinal reflex or not eliciting a response if a spinal cord injury is present.

Comprehensive Neurologic Assessment

COMPONENT	POSSIBLE FINDINGS
Level of consciousness	Orientation Hypoarousal: lethargy, obtunded, stupor Hyperarousal: restlessness, agitation Language: dysphasia, dysarthria Mentation: memory, attention
Pupillary assessment	Examination: size, shape, response to light, consensual Abnormal pupils: unilateral fixed and dilated, bilateral fixed and dilated, pinpoint

Comprehensive Neurologic Assessment (continued)

COMPONENT	POSSIBLE FINDINGS
Brain stem reflexes	Corneals Extraocular movements: doll's eyes (oculocephalic reflex), caloric (oculovestibular reflex), gaze, tracking Cough Gag

Focal/localizing signs	Glasgow Coma Scale: motor
	  6, Follows commands
	  5, Localizes to pain (purposeful)
	  4, Normal flexion (withdrawal)
	  3, Abnormal flexion (decortication)
	  2, Extension (decerebration)
	  1, None
	Pronator drift
	Muscle strength
	  5, normal power
	  4, moves against gravity with some resistance
	  3, moves against gravity without resistance
	  2, moves without gravity
	  1, flicker of movement
	  0, no movement
	Facial droop

External signs of head injury	Bruises, lacerations, abrasions
Vital signs	Respirations: Cheyne-Stokes respirations, central neurogenic hyperventilation, apneustic, ataxic Heart rate: sinus tachycardia, bradycardia Blood pressure: hypertension, hypotension
Preexisting conditions	Head injury, stroke, peripheral nerve injury, spinal cord injury, Parkinson's disease, cardiac disease, pulmonary disease, other

Guidelines for Management of Severe Head Injury

STANDARD	GUIDELINE	OPTIONAL
Chronic prophylactic hyper-ventilation should be avoided in absence of IICP during first 5 days	All areas of United States should have organized trauma system	Neurosurgeons should have an organized plan to care for neurotrauma
Barbiturate therapy should be considered for refractory IICP if hemodynamically stable	Avoid hypotension and hypoxia	Priority of treatment: complete fluid resuscitation. No treatment for IICP unless signs of herniation
Glucocorticoids are not recom-mended in severe head injury	ICP monitoring appropriate for Glasgow Coma Scale 3–8 with abnormal CT scan, or with 2 or more of the following: age >40 yrs, motor posturing, blood pressure ≤90 mm Hg	Mean SABP should be maintained >90 mm Hg

Prophylactic anticonvulsants (phenytoin, carbamazepine, phenobarbital) are not recommended for preventing late posttraumatic seizures	ICP treatment threshold 20–25 mm Hg. Treatment for ICP should be corroborated by clinical examination	Cerebral perfusion pressure should be maintained at a minimum of 70 mm Hg
	Prophylactic hyperventilation should be avoided during the first 24 hr	Brief hyperventilation may be necessary to treat acute neurologic deterioration or longer for refractory IICP
	Mannitol is effective to treat IICP. Bolus better than continuous infusion	Use of mannitol without ICP monitoring is indicated with signs of herniation or neurologic deterioration. Maintain euvolemia, serum osmolarity < 320 mOsm
		Preferable feeding method is gastrojejunostomy
	Nutritional replacement: 140% resting metabolism expenditure if nonparalyzed, 100% if paralyzed	
		Early posttraumatic seizures may be treated with phenytoin or carbamazepine or no treatment may be given. Does not appear to affect outcome

ICP, intracranial pressure; IICP, increased intracranial pressure; SABP, systemic arterial blood pressure.

Pharmacologic Management of Increased Intracranial Pressure

DRUG	DOSE RANGE	MECHANISM OF ACTION	SPECIAL CONSIDERATIONS
Sedatives			
Midazolam	0.01–0.1 mg/kg IV	Sedative, hypnotic, anxiolytic, amnesic, skeletal muscle relaxant, anticonvulsant	Respiratory and cardiac depression
Lorazepam	0.01–0.06 mg/kg IM/IV		
Diazepam	1–10 mg IV		
Propofol	5–50 μg/kg/min or greater	Sedative, hypnotic	May produce hemodynamic instability and respiratory depression
			Tubing and solution should be changed every 12 hr
			Rapid onset and elimination, allowing assessment. Slowly wean continuous infusions
			Expensive
Haloperidol	0.03–0.07 mg/kg IM/IV	Central antidopaminergic, weak anticholinergic	Extrapyramidal symptoms—rigidity
Morphine sulfate	1–10 mg IV	Analgesic	Respiratory depression
Short-acting paralytics			
Pancuronium bromide	0.1 mg/kg IV	Neuromuscular blocking agents	Must be intubated. May be given in intermittent bolus or infusion; will affect neurologic examination
Vecuronium	0.1 mg/kg		
Atracurium	0.4–0.5 mg/kg		

Lidocaine	1–1.5 mg/kg IV or intratracheal	Stabilizes cell membrane, blunts cough	Monitor cardiac rhythm
Mannitol	0.25–1 g/kg IV	Osmotic diuretic, decreases CSF production, changes rheology of RBCs	Best response with bolus administration. Avoid dehydration—keep serum osmolarity less than 315–320 mOsm.
Furosemide	0.5–1 mg/kg IV 0.15–0.3 mg/kg if given with mannitol	Loop diuretic, decreases CSF production	Avoid dehydration.
Barbiturates Pentobarbital	10 mg/kg over 30 min 5 mg/kg × 3 hr, followed by 1–2 mg/kg/hr	Suppresses neuronal activity, stabilizes cell membranes Decreases CBF, $CMRO_2$, and glucose utilization	Suppresses cardiovascular and immune systems. Keep hydrated. Support with vasopressors. Consider PA catheter. Monitor levels (3–4 mg/dL)
Thiopental	5–11 mg/kg over 15–30 min 4–8 mg/kg/hr		

IV, intravenously; IM, intramuscularly; CBF, cerebral blood flow; $CMRO_2$, cerebral metabolic rate of oxygen; CSF, cerebrospinal fluid; RBC, red blood cell; PA, pulmonary artery.

Signs and Symptoms of Herniation

CINGULATE	UNCAL	CENTRAL	INFRATENTORIAL
Lateral displacement of the cingulate gyrus under falx cerebri	Lateral and downward displacement of the temporal lobe through the tentorium incisura	Downward displacement of the cerebrum and diencephalon onto the brain stem	Downward displacement of the brain stem through the foramen magnum
Decreased LOC	Early: altered LOC, ipsilateral pupil dilation, disconjugate doll's eyes, contralateral motor weakness	Early: altered LOC, Cheyne-Stokes respiration, small pupils, localization of noxious stimuli, intact doll's eyes	Precipitous increase in SABP, small pupils, disconjugate gaze, ataxic respirations, quadriparesis

Late: central neurogenic hyperventilation or Cheyne-Stokes
respiration, ipsilateral fixed and
dilated pupil, disconjugate
doll's eye, contralateral decortication or decerebration

Late diencephalon: altered LOC,
Cheyne-Stokes respiration, small
pupils, decortication, intact doll's
eyes

Midbrain, upper pons: coma, central
neurogenic hyperventilation, fixed
midposition, irregular pupils, disconjugate doll's eyes, decerebrate

Pons, upper medulla: coma, ataxic respiration, dilated fixed pupils, flaccid,
lower extremities—triple flexion

LOC, level of consciousness; SABP, systemic arterial blood pressure.

Progression and Signs and Symptoms With Herniation

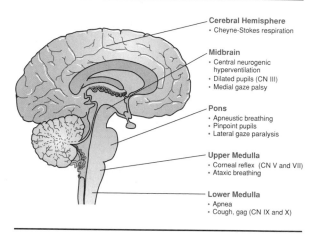

Cerebral Hemisphere
- Cheyne-Stokes respiration

Midbrain
- Central neurogenic hyperventilation
- Dilated pupils (CN III)
- Medial gaze palsy

Pons
- Apneustic breathing
- Pinpoint pupils
- Lateral gaze paralysis

Upper Medulla
- Corneal reflex (CN V and VII)
- Ataxic breathing

Lower Medulla
- Apnea
- Cough, gag (CN IX and X)

37

Spinal Cord Injury

Levels of Injury and Expected Functional Ability

CERVICAL LEVEL OF INJURY	NORMAL FUNCTION	EXPECTED FUNCTION
C1–C2	Head and neck control Respiratory muscle control Shoulder shrug	Limited movement of the head and neck Ventilator dependent Electric wheelchair with breath or head control Dependent in all ADLs Use of mouthstick to type, write, or turn pages
C3–C4	Mouth control Shoulder/scapular movement Diaphragm movement	Good head and neck control May or may not be ventilator dependent but will need ventilator support acutely Dependent in all ADLs Electric wheelchair with breath, head, or shoulder controls

Level		
C5	Shoulder flexion Elbow flexion Increased scapular function	Full head, neck, shoulder, and diaphragm control Can assist in ADLs, but still requires major assistance Can feed self with special assistive devices Able to move wheelchair for short distances, but does better with an electric wheelchair
C6	Good wrist flexion Wrist extension Shoulder rotation and abduction	Independent in feeding and some grooming with assistive devices Can roll over in bed Requires minor assistance in transfer Can drive a car with hand controls
C7	Elbow extension Strong wrist extension Shoulder full movement Some finger control	Transfers independently Independent in most ADLs Excellent bed mobility
C8–T1	Normal hand strength	Bed and wheelchair independent

ADLs, activities of daily living.

Standard Neurologic Classification of Spinal Cord Injury

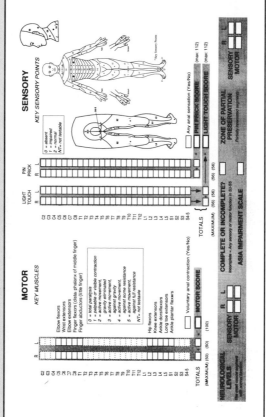

From *International Standards for Neurological and Functional Classification of Spinal Cord Injury.* With permission from the American Spinal Injury Association, Atlanta, GA. 1996.

Functional Independence Measures (FIM)

LEVELS		
7 Complete independence (timely, safely) 6 Modified independence (device)		No helper
Modified Dependence 5 Supervision 4 Minimal assist (subject = 75%+) 3 Moderate assist (subject = 50%+) **Complete Dependence** 2 Maximal assist (subject = 25%+) 1 Total assist (subject = 0%+)		Helper

	Self-Care	Admit	Discharge
A.	Eating	☐	☐
B.	Grooming	☐	☐
C.	Bathing	☐	☐
D.	Dressing, upper body	☐	☐
E.	Dressing, lower body	☐	☐
F.	Toileting	☐	☐
	Sphincter Control		
G.	Bladder management	☐	☐
H.	Bowel management	☐	☐
	Mobility		
	Transfer:		
I.	Bed, chair, wheelchair	☐	☐
J.	Toilet	☐	☐
K.	Tub, shower	☐	☐
	Locomotion	W☐	W☐
L.	Walk/wheelchair	C☐	C☐
M.	Stairs	☐	☐
	Communication	A☐	A☐
N.	Comprehension	V☐	V☐
O.	Expression	V☐ N☐	V☐ N☐
	Social Cognition		
P.	Social interaction	☐	☐
Q.	Problem solving	☐	☐
R.	Memory	☐	☐
	Total FIM	☐	☐

NOTE: Leave no blanks; enter 1 if patient not testable due to risk

American Spinal Injury Association Impairment Scale

☐ **A. = Complete:** No motor or sensory function is preserved in the sacral segments S4-S5.

☐ **B. = Incomplete:** Sensory but not motor function is preserved below the neurologic level and extends through the sacral segments S4-S5.

☐ **C. = Incomplete:** Motor function is preserved below the neurologic level, and the majority of key muscles below the neurologic level have a muscle grade less than 3.

☐ **D. = Incomplete:** Motor function is preserved below the neurologic level, and the majority of key muscles below the neurologic level have a muscle grade greater than or equal to 3.

☐ **E. = Normal:** Motor and sensory function are normal.

CLINICAL SYNDROMES

☐ Central cord

☐ Brown-Séquard

☐ Anterior cord

☐ Conus medullaris

☐ Cauda equina

Potential Causes and Clinical Manifestations of Autonomic Dysreflexia

Potential Causes

Overdistended bladder
Distended bowel
Skin breakdown
Excessive skin stimulation
Excessive skin pressure
Sudden change in environmental temperature
Infection
Pain

Clinical Manifestations

Hypertension
Triggering of a vagal response
Bradycardia
Severe headache
Diaphoresis and flushing above the level of the lesion
Coolness and pallor below the level of the lesion

38

Guillain-Barré Syndrome

Signs of Autonomic System Involvement in Guillain-Barré Syndrome

SYSTEM	SIGNS AND SYMPTOMS
Cardiac	Dysrhythmias, particularly tachydysrhythmias Labile blood pressure Hypertension Hypotension Abnormal hemodynamic response to drugs
Neurologic	Pupillary dysfunction
Gastrointestinal	Constipation
Genitourinary	Retention
Integument	Flushing and sweating

Cranial Nerves Commonly Affected in Guillain-Barré Syndrome

CRANIAL NERVE		MOTOR FUNCTION
III	Oculomotor	Elevation of eyelids Extraocular movement
IV	Trochlear	Extraocular movement (downward and inward)
VI	Abducens	Extraocular movement (outward)
VII	Facial	Facial expressions
IX	Glossopharyngeal	Swallowing
X	Vagus	Swallowing, gag reflex

39

Cerebrovascular Disorders

Risk Factors Associated With the Development of Stroke

Hypertension
Smoking
Obesity
Drug and alcohol abuse
Sedentary life style
Hyperlipidemia
Atrial fibrillation
Left ventricular hypertrophy
Heart failure
Ischemic heart disease
History of transient ischemic attacks
Diabetes
Elevated hematocrit levels

Metabolic Cascade That Leads to Cell Death

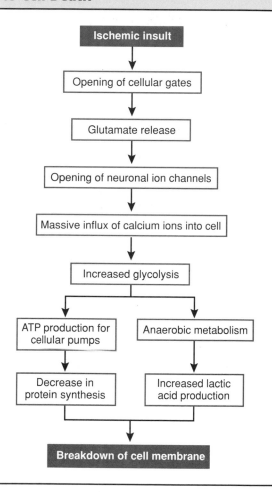

Incidence of Intracranial Aneurysms by Arterial Distribution

INTRACRANIAL ARTERY	INCIDENCE
Cavernous segment internal carotid artery (ICA)	5%
Supraclinoid ICA (includes supraclinoid segment of ICA, ophthalmic artery, posterior communicating artery, and anterior choroidal artery)	24–40%
Anterior cerebral artery and anterior communicating artery	33%
Middle cerebral artery	21–31%
Vertebrobasilar system	5–12%

From *AACN Clinical Reference Guide for Critical-Care Nursing.* St. Louis, Mosby–Year Book, Inc.

Clinical Findings Associated With Stroke by Arterial Distribution*

ARTERIAL DISTRIBUTION	POSSIBLE CLINICAL FINDINGS

Anterior
  Anterior cerebral artery
  Middle cerebral artery
  Internal carotid artery
	Contralateral hemiparesis
	Contralateral sensory deficits
	Aphasias (left-sided lesions in left cerebral dominance)
	Dysphagia
	Altered mental status
	Post-stroke depression
	Unilateral neglect (visual and/or tactile; more common with right cerebral infarction)
	Gaze preference
	Apraxia
	Signs and symptoms of increased intracranial pressure when size of lesion produces mass effect

(continued)

Clinical Findings Associated With Stroke by Arterial Distribution* (continued)

ARTERIAL DISTRIBUTION	POSSIBLE CLINICAL FINDINGS
Posterior 　Vertebrobasilar system 　Posterior cerebral artery	Dysphagia Ataxia Visual field defects Gaze preference/ disconjugate extraocular movements Nystagmus Motor and sensory deficits, including bilateral hemiparesis Altered level of consciousness Signs and symptoms of increased intracranial pressure when size of lesion produces mass effect

*Clinical signs and symptoms vary according to precise location of the stroke within the brain.

Grade of Subarachnoid Hemorrhage and Associated Outcomes

HUNT AND HESS SCALE

Grade	Neurologic Status
I	Asymptomatic or minimal headache and slight nuchal rigidity
II	Moderate to severe headache, meningismus, no neurologic deficit other than cranial nerve palsy
III	Drowsiness, confusion, minimal focal neurologic deficit
IV	Stuporous, moderate to severe hemiparesis, possible early decerebrate rigidity and vegetative disturbances
V	Deep coma, decerebrate posturing, moribund appearance

GLASGOW OUTCOME SCALE

Category	Outcome
1	Good recovery, independent lifestyle
2	Moderate disability, independent lifestyle
3	Severe disability, conscious but not independent
4	Vegetative
5	Dead

Adapted from the work of Hunt WE, Hess RM: Surgical risk as related to time of intervention in the repair of intracranial aneurysms. *J Neurosurg* 28:14–20, 1968; Mendel RC, Carter LP: Evaluation and treatment of clinical vasospasm following subarachnoid hemorrhage. *Contemp Neurosurg* 16(6):1–6, 1994; Findley JM: Perioperative management of subarachnoid hemorrhage. *Contemp Neurosurg* 17(6):1–5, 1995; National Stroke Association: Management of subarachnoid hemorrhage. *Stroke Clin Updates* 6(1):1–4, 1995. Reprinted from AACN Clinical Reference Guide for Critical-Care Nursing. St. Louis, Mosby–Year Book, Inc.

The Spetzler and Martin Arteriovenous Malformation (AVM) Grading System

CRITERIA	CORRESPONDING SCORE
Size of AVM nidus	AVM score by size
Small: < 3 cm	Small: 1
Medium: 3–6 cm	Medium: 2
Large: > 6 cm	Large: 3
Eloquence of adjacent brain	AVM score by eloquence
Noneloquent	0
Eloquent	1
Deep vascular component	AVM score by vascular depth
Limited to superficial	0
Deep component present	1
Sum of AVM scores = total score or AVM grade	

Brain eloquence is defined as a region of the brain that harbors easily identifiable neurologic function that if injured would result in disabling neurologic deficit. The Spetzler and Martin system has demonstrated the highest overall correlation with operative difficulty and postoperative neurologic outcome. Adapted from the work of Spetzler RF, Martin NA: A proposed grading system for arteriovenous malformations. *J Neurosurg* 65:476–483, 1986. From AACN Clinical Reference Guide for Critical-Care Nursing. St. Louis, Mosby–Year Book, Inc.

Criteria for the Diagnosis of Vasospasm by Transcranial Doppler

MEAN MIDDLE CEREBRAL ARTERY VELOCITY (MCAV)	DEGREE OF VASOSPASM
100–120 cm/sec	Borderline
120–160 cm/sec	Mild
160–200 cm/sec	Moderate
>200 cm/sec	Severe

From AACN Clinical Reference Guide for Critical-Care Nursing. St. Louis, Mosby–Year Book, Inc.

Pentobarbital Coma Protocol

1. Anesthesia consult: intubation, oximetric pulmonary artery catheter insertion, jugular bulb catheter insertion, and initiation of pentobarbital protocol
2. Clinical pharmacist consult for ongoing medication/interaction monitoring
3. Registered dietitian consult for comprehensive enteral nutritional support
4. Ventilator and intubation setup to bedside
5. Place warming blanket on bed; continuous temperature monitoring and automatic blanket temperature adjustments to maintain patient temperature between 97° and 100° F.
6. a. Administer loading dose of pentobarbital 10 mg/kg over 30 min IV
   b. Follow with pentobarbital 5 mg/kg/hr × 3 hr to achieve a serum pentobarbital concentration >2 mg/dL
   c. Follow with a maintenance dose of 2.5 mg/kg/hr
   d. If intracranial pressure increases above 20 mm Hg, and the serum pentobarbital concentration is <3 mg/dL, administer an additional pentobarbital 5 mg/kg IV over 30 min to reduce the pressure
7. Administer morphine sulfate _____ mg IV q2hr for duration of pentobarbital therapy

8. Administer _____ (paralytic agent) ____ mg IV _____ (frequency) for duration of pentobarbital therapy; assess depth of neuromuscular blockade every 15 minutes until 1–2 twitch response is achieved; follow with assessments every 8 hours of depth of neuromuscular blockade

9. Obtain baseline arterial blood gas levels, hematocrit and hemoglobin, serum osmolarity, and cardiac output with calculated hemodynamic profile within 1 hour of loading dose administration

10. Draw serum pentobarbital levels at 4, 8, 12, and 24 hours after initial loading dose administered (therapeutic range = 2–4 mg/dL)

11. Continuous SvO_2, SpO_2, JvO_2, and temperature monitoring

12. Repeat cardiac output every 8 hours for first 24 hours, then once a day and as needed for duration of pentobarbital therapy

13. Serum pentobarbital levels once a day for duration of therapy; maintain level between 2 and 4 mg/dL

14. Set ventricular drain at an overflow level of ____ mm Hg/cm H_2O; document intracranial pressure, cerebral perfusion pressure, and ventricular drainage hourly

---

Adapted with permission from the Health Outcomes Institute, Inc., The Woodlands, TX.

Clinical Findings Associated With Tube Feeding Dependency Following Stroke

Wet voice after swallowing water
Cough during or immediately after water swallow
Hypoglossal nerve dysfunction
Incomplete oral closure

Adapted from Wojner AW, Walton MW, Dildy T, Newmark M: Predictors of tube feeding dependency following acute stroke. In press.

Recombinant Tissue Plasminogen Activator Ischemic Stroke Inclusion/Exclusion Criteria Checklist

Inclusion Criteria

_____ Age ≥ 18 years and functionally independent before current presentation

_____ Clinical diagnosis of ischemic stroke with measurable neurologic deficit

_____ Computed tomography (CT) scan negative for intracranial hemorrhage

_____ Presentation within 180 min of symptom onset

Exclusion Criteria

_____ Rapid improvement in neurologic function prior to treatment

_____ CT scan positive for intracranial hemorrhage

_____ Evolving infarction documented on CT scan with acute hypodensity or mass effect

_____ Presentation suggests subarachnoid hemorrhage in the face of a negative CT

_____ History of seizure prior to or during stroke event

_____ Extreme moribund presentation

_____ Inability to maintain systolic blood pressure < 185 or diastolic blood pressure < 110 mm Hg

_____ Aggressive hypertension control requiring sodium nitroprusside

_____ Serum glucose < 50 mg/dL or > 400 mg/dL

_____ History of surgery or trauma within the past 14 days

_____ Arterial puncture at a noncompressible site

_____ Lumbar puncture within the past 7 days

_____ History positive for stroke within the last 3 months

_____ History of intracranial hemorrhage

_____ Possible postmyocardial pericarditis

_____ Lactating or pregnant female

Reprinted with permission from the Health Outcomes Institute, Inc., The Woodlands, TX.

Recombinant Tissue Plasminogen Activator (rtPA) Ischemic Stroke Order Set

1. Complete inclusion/exclusion criteria checklist
2. Call stroke response team STAT
3. Start 2 IV lines as follows
   a. Dedicated rtPA infusion line
   b. Keep vein open line for other fluid and medication administration
5. Insert Foley catheter if patient unable to void prior to start of rtPA infusion
6. Calculate dosage of rtPA 0.9 mg/kg:
   Step A. Patient weight _____ kg × 0.9 mg = _____ **mg total rtPA dose**
   (*Stop: Check dose;* if greater than 90 mg by calculation, give total of 90 mg only)
   Step B. Administer 10% of total rtPA dose as an initial bolus:
   _____ mg total rtPA dose × 0.10 = _____ **mg bolus dose**
   Step C. Administer the balance of the rtPA over the next 60 min:
   _____ mg total rtPA − _____ mg bolus dose = _____ **mg infusion dose**
7. Neurologic vital signs q15 min for 1 hour; then begin q1 hr for 5 hr, and then q2 hr for 18 hr. Increase frequency of neurologic vital signs as indicated by patient's clinical status. Notify physician STAT of signs and symptoms of deterioration
8. Cardiac monitoring for 24 hr
9. *Following rtPA infusion,* no nasoenteric/nasogastric tube insertions, Foley catheter insertions, or invasive lines/procedures for 24 hr unless clinically indicated
10. STAT brain computed tomography for signs and symptoms of clinical deterioration
11. Stop anticoagulant or antiplatelet medications until further notice

Adapted with permission from the Health Outcomes Institute, Inc., The Woodlands, TX.

40

Seizure Disorders

Factors Associated With Increased Risk for Epilepsy

Family history of epilepsy or febrile seizures
Perinatal injuries such as toxemia during pregnancy, delivery problems, neonatal hypoxia/anoxia, low birth weight
Toxic and metabolic disturbances
Stroke
Anoxia
Craniocerebral trauma
Central nervous system infections such as viral encephalitis and bacterial and aseptic meningitis
Congenital cerebral malformations
Subarachnoid hemorrhage and vasospasm
Use of and withdrawal from alcohol and drugs
Alzheimer's disease
Multiple sclerosis
Tumors
Abrupt withdrawal of antiepileptic medications or chronically used sedatives

Medications That May Lower the Seizure Threshold

DRUG CLASSIFICATION	EXAMPLES
ANTIDEPRESSANTS	Imipramine, amitriptyline, doxepin, nortriptyline, maprotiline, mianserin, nomifensine, bupropion
ANTIPSYCHOTICS	Chlorpromazine, thioridazine, perphenazine, trifluoperazine, prochlorperazine, haloperidol
ANALGESICS	Fentanyl, meperidine, pentazocine, propoxyphene, cocaine, mefenamic acid, tramadol
LOCAL ANESTHETICS	Lidocaine, mepivacaine, procaine, bupivacaine, etidocaine

(continued)

Medications That May Lower the Seizure Threshold (continued)

DRUG CLASSIFICATION	EXAMPLES
GENERAL ANESTHETICS	Ketamine, halothane, enflurane, propanidid, methohexital
ANTIMICROBIALS	Penicillin, synthetic penicillins (oxacillin, carbenicillin, ticarcillin), ampicillin, cephalosporins, metronidazole, nalidixic acid, isoniazid, cycloserine, pyrimethamine, imipenem
ANTINEOPLASTICS	Chlorambucil, vincristine, methotrexate, cytosine arabinoside, misonidazole, BCNU, PALA, busulfan
BRONCHODILATORS	Aminophylline, theophylline
SYMPATHOMIMETICS	Ephedrine, terbutaline, phenylpropanolamine
OTHER	Insulin, antihistamines, anticholinergics, baclofen, cyclosporin A, lithium, atenolol, disopyramide, phencyclidine, amphetamines, domperidone, doxapram, ergonovine, folic acid, camphor, methylxanthines, thyrotropin-releasing hormone, vitamin K oxide, aqueous iodinated contrast media, oxytocin, hyperosmolar parenteral solutions, hyperbaric oxygen, antiepileptic medications, methylphenidate, flumazenil

Adapted from Mastaglia FL: Iatrogenic (drug-induced) disorders of the nervous system. In Aminoff MJ (ed): The Neurological Aspects of Medical Disorders. New York, Churchill Livingstone, 1989; and Boggs, 1989.

Examples of Conditions Contributing to Development of Seizure Activity

Atrial fibrillation
Subacute bacterial endocarditis
Altered protein binding
Dysequilibrium syndrome
HIV-positive status
Intracranial structural lesions
Cerebral aneurysm rupture
Cardiac/respiratory arrest
Uremia
Primary central nervous system infections
Neurocysticercosis
Immunosuppression

From Boggs JG: Seizures in medically complex patients. Epilepsia 38(suppl 4):555–559, 1997.

International Classification of Seizures

CLASSIFICATION	SUBCLASSIFICATION	ASSOCIATED SYMPTOMS
Partial (focal) seizures	Simple partial (without impairment or loss of consciousness)	Motor signs
		Somatosensory or special sensory symptoms
		Autonomic symptoms or signs
		Psychic symptoms
		Simple partial onset, with progression to complex partial onset with impairment of consciousness
	Complex partial (with impairment or loss of consciousness)	Simple partial with secondary generalization
	Partial seizures with secondary generalization	Complex partial with secondary generalization
		Simple partial to complex partial with secondary generalization

Generalized	Tonic-clonic	Initiated tonic phase associated with rigidity Clonic phase follows and is associated with rhythmic jerking activity
	Absence	Blank stare, rapid eye blinking May go unnoticed
	Myoclonic	Brief massive muscle jerks
	Atonic	Sudden loss of muscle tone and consciousness Also known as "drop attacks"
	Tonic only	Rigidity of all or parts of body
	Clonic only	Rhythmic jerking movements
Unclassified		Seizures that do not meet any of the above criteria; often seen in neonates

Adapted from Commission on Classification and Terminology of the International League Against Epilepsy: Proposed for revised clinical and electroencephalographic classification of epileptic seizures. Epilepsia 22:489–501, 1981.

Safety Measures During a Seizure

Remove harmful objects from the environment
Support the patient's head
Stay with the patient during the seizure
Gently guide the patient to positions of safety
Do not restrain the patient
Insertion of a tongue blade is currently controversial
    (could damage the oral cavity if forced inside)
Monitor blood pressure and heart rate closely during
    and following the seizure

Components of a Health History Following a Seizure

CATEGORY	TOPICS TO EXPLORE
Detailed description of the event(s)	Occurrences before the seizure activity took place
	Initial onset of symptoms, including prodrome or aura
	Progression of the seizure activity
	What happened during the postictal period
Medical history	Past history of seizures, including febrile convulsions
	Predisposing factors such as head trauma, stroke, substance abuse, or infections
Family history	Febrile seizures
	Seizure history in parents, siblings, and immediate family
	Other neurologic disorders in the family
Psychosocial history	Coping patterns
	Discrimination
	Social exclusion
	Negative life events
	Stigma
	Support systems
	Occupation
	Recent travel

Data from Ellis C: Nursing assessment and intervention for the patient experiencing seizures: a structured approach. Clin Nurs Pract Epilepsy 1(2):4–7, 1993; and Leppik IE: Contemporary Diagnosis and Management of the Patient With Epilepsy, 3rd ed. Newtown, PA: Handbooks in Health Care, 1997.

The Spectrum of the Effects of Epilepsy

CATEGORY	DESCRIPTIONS
Uncomplicated	Majority in this category Seizures controlled with medications Minimal side effects Well-established support system Rare academic, vocational, or psychological problems
Compromised	Seizures usually controlled Can have fluctuating difficulties in social, emotional, cognitive, and functional domains, quality of life Can have altered health perceptions Without in-depth assessment, appear well adapted
Devastated	Multiple problems, including impaired learning and motor and emotional functioning Seizures often never controlled May have associated cognitive dysfunction related to the underlying brain disease Support system stressed, with altered coping Epilepsy may be the focus of a family's life Require continuous intervention and reassurement

Data from Santilli N: The spectrum of epilepsy. Clin Nurs Pract Epilepsy 1:4–7, 1993; and Marshall RH, Capoli JM: Epilepsy and education: the pediatrician's expanding role. Adv Pediatr 33:159–180, 1996.

The Major Drugs Used To Treat Status Epilepticus

	DIAZEPAM	LORAZEPAM	FOSPHENYTOIN	PHENOBARBITAL
Adult IV dose (mg/kg)	0.15–0.25	0.1	15–20 phenytoin equiv	20
Maximal administration rate (mg/min)	5	2.0	150 phenytoin equiv	20
Minutes to cessation of convulsive status epilepticus	1–3	6–10	10–30	20–30
Duration of action (hr)	0.25–0.5	>12–24	24	>48
Elimination half-life (hr)	30	24	24	100
Volume of distribution (L/kg)	1–2	0.7–1.0	0.5–0.8	0.7
Potential side effects				
Depression of consciousness	10–30 min	Several hours	None	Several days
Respiratory depression	Occasional	Occasional	Infrequent	Occasional
Hypotension	Infrequent	Infrequent	Occasional	Infrequent
Cardiac arrhythmias	—	—	In patients with heart disease	—

Data from Epilepsy Foundation of America's Working Group on Status Epilepticus: Treatment of convulsive status epilepticus. JAMA 270:845–859, 1993; Treiman DM: General principles of treatment: Response and intractable status epilepticus in adults. Adv Neurol 34:377–384, 1983; Treiman DM: Special treatment problems in adults. In Smith DB (ed): Epilepsy: Current Approaches to Diagnosis and Treatment, New York, Raven Press, 1990, pp 155–172.

Common Medications Used To Treat Epilepsy

DRUG	USUAL MAXIMUM ADULT DOSAGE	TIME TO STEADY STATE	HALF-LIFE	ELIMINATION	THERA-PEUTIC RANGE	COMMON SIDE EFFECTS	AFFECTED BY ANTI-EPILEPTIC DRUG	AFFECT ANTI-EPILEPTIC DRUG
Carbamazepine (CBZ;	400–2400 mg/day BID–QID	4–6 wk; after induction, 2–4 days	8–72 hr	1–3% unchanged in urine	4–14 mL	Dizziness, diplopia, drowsiness, blurred and double vision, nausea, headache, leukopenia	Oral contraceptives, warfarin, theophylline, doxycycline	Fluoxetine, propoxyphene, erythromycin, cimetidine, felbamate, phenobarbital, PHT
Felbamate (FBM;	3600 mg/day TID–QID	5–7 days	20–23 hr	50–60% metabolized; 40–60% unchanged in urine	Not defined	Anorexia, weight loss, vomiting, insomnia, nausea, headache, aplastic anemia,* hepatic failure*	PHT, VPA, CBZ and its epoxide	PHT, CBZ, VPA

(continued)

457

Common Medications Used To Treat Epilepsy (continued)

DRUG	USUAL MAXIMUM ADULT DOSAGE	TIME TO STEADY STATE	HALF-LIFE	ELIMINATION	THERA-PEUTIC RANGE	COMMON SIDE EFFECTS	AFFECTED BY ANTI-EPILEPTIC DRUG	AFFECT ANTI-EPILEPTIC DRUG
Gabapentin (GBP)	4800 mg/day TID-QID	Renal function dependent; 1–2 days normal renal function	5–7 hr with normal function; up to 132 hr with anuria	Renal; not metabolized	Not defined	Fatigue, somnolence, weight gain, dizziness, ataxia	None	Aluminum hydroxide, magnesium hydroxide

Lamotrigine (LTG)[a]	100–150 mg/day with VPA; 300–500 mg/day without VPA; BID–TID	3–15 days	Varies depending on monotherapy, presence of other enzyme inducers, VPA range	85% metabolized in liver; 10% unchanged in urine	Not defined	Drowsiness, headache, tremor, diplopia, ataxia, abnormal thinking, nervousness, weight gain, nausea, vomiting	CBZ, epoxide, VPA	PHT, CBZ, phenobarbital, primidone, VPA

PHT, phenytoin; VPA, valproic acid.

[a] Felbamate should be used only in situations in which risk is fully weighed and is clearly understood by patient and family because of the high incidence of these side effects.

Data from Leppik IE, Wolff D: Antiepileptic medication interaction. Neurol Clin 2:905–921, 1993; and Levy RH, Meldrum BS (eds): Antiepileptic Drugs. 4th ed. New York, Raven Press, 1995.

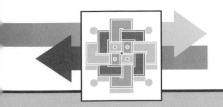

Multisystem
Disorders

41

Consequences of Immunodeficiency

Comparison of Serologic Tests for HIV Infection

TEST	DESCRIPTION
Enzyme-linked immunosorbent assay (HIV-1 ELISA)	Usually the first test performed on a blood sample to identify if a person is negative or positive for HIV antibodies. A sensitive, though nonspecific test, ELISA must be confirmed by Western blot. False-negative tests may result if the person is tested during the window period. Most variants except subtype O are detected by this test. There is a combined HIV-1/HIV-2 test on the market, which is used by the blood banks in the United States. Average cost is $20.00
Immunofluorescence assay (IFA)	A confirmatory test that uses a fluorescent dye to determine the presence of HIV antibodies
Western blot (WB)	Used to verify the ELISA findings. An antibody test, it uses the protein bands of the virus to test against
Polymerase chain reaction (PCR)	Unlike the antibody test, PCR searches for viral DNA attached to host DNA inside the nucleus of the cell
p24 antigen	A specific protein found in the core of the virus that signifies rapid replication of the virus. Increased p24 antigen levels occur twice during viral replication, shortly after the initial infection and again when the patient reaches the AIDS designation whereby the immune system is overpowered and unable to produce significant antibodies to fight the production of HIV
OraSure (an oral transudate test for HIV-1)	Has the same sensitivity as ELISA, but is easier to collect. Must also be confirmed by Western blot. Patients place a collection pad (looks like a small toothbrush) between their lower gum and cheek for 2–5 min. Fluid (oral mucosal transudate), which may contain antibodies to HIV, is drawn through the cheek and gums onto the pad. The device is then removed and placed into a small vial containing a preservative and sent to the laboratory for analysis

Opportunistic Diseases Found in Patients with HIV Infection

ORGANISM/VIRUS	CLINICAL PRESENTATION	CURRENT TREATMENT STRATEGIES
Cytomegalovirus (CMV)	CMV retinitis (loss of visual field, blurred vision) Pneumonitis (usually seen with other infections like *Pneumocystis carinii* pneumonia or *Mycobacterium avium* complex infection, progressive shortness of breath, dyspnea on exertion, dry nonproductive cough with or without fever) Encephalitis (personality changes, cognitive impairment, motor impairment) Colitis (weight loss, anorexia, fever) Esophagitis (ulcers) Adrenalitis (postural hypotension and sodium deficits)	Ganciclovir Foscarnet Colony-stimulating factor (investigational)
HIV encephalopathy (AIDS dementia complex)	Inability to concentrate, decreased memory, slowness in thinking, leg weakness, ataxia, clumsiness, apathy, reduced spontaneity, social withdrawal, irritability, hyperactivity, anxiety without an identifiable cause, mania, delirium, euphoria, grandiose delusions	Zidovudine Didanosine Methylphenidate Dextroamphetamine

Herpes simplex virus (HSV) disease	Oral lesions (ulcers on lips, tongue, pharynx, or buccal mucosa; fever; pharyngitis; cervical lymphadenopathy) Genital lesions (inguinal lymphadenopathy, dysuria) Perianal and anorectal lesions (localized pain, itching, pain on defecation, tenesmus, constipation, sacral radiculopathy, impotence, neurogenic bladder) HSV esophagitis (dysphagia, odynophagia, and retrosternal pain) HSV encephalitis (headache, meningismus, personality change, fever, nausea, lethargy, confusion, cranial nerve deficits, and seizures)	Acyclovir (intravenous, oral, or topical) Foscarnet for acyclovir-resistant HSV-2 infection
Lymphoma, Non-Hodgkin's (NHL)	Nonspecific symptoms, unexplained fever, drenching night sweats, or weight loss greater than 10% of total body weight; confusion, lethargy, memory loss, hemiparesis, aphasia, seizures, cranial nerve palsies, headache, numbness of the chin, and stiff neck	Standard dose chemotherapy for those with good immune function and no previous opportunistic infections. Lower dose chemotherapy for immunocompromised patients, history of opportunistic infections. Regimens using chemotherapy, antiretrovirals, prophylaxis for *Pneumocystis carinii* pneumonia and colony-stimulating factor under investigation *(continued)*

Opportunistic Diseases Found in Patients with HIV Infection (continued)

ORGANISM/VIRUS	CLINICAL PRESENTATION	CURRENT TREATMENT STRATEGIES
Recurrent pneumonia	Abrupt onset with fever, cough with purulent sputum, and systemic toxic effects	Broad-spectrum antimicrobial therapy until organism identified, then change to appropriate antibiotic. Additional treatment measures: fluids, antipyretic drugs, airway suction or postural drainage, bronchodilator for bronchospasm
Progressive multifocal leukoencephalopathy (PML)	Extremity weakness, cognitive dysfunction, visual loss, gait disturbances, limb incoordination, headache, speech or language disturbance, spastic hemiparesis, visual field loss, altered mentation. Cerebellar involvement: ataxia, limb dysmetria, dysarthria. Cortical infection: aphasia, apraxia, Gerstmann's syndrome, prosopagnosia, left-sided neglect, and impaired spatial orientation	No form of therapy for PML has been effective
Salmonellosis	Fever, chills, sweats, weight loss, diarrhea, and anorexia	Ampicillin and chloramphenicol are the most often used third-generation cephalosporins, amoxicillin, ciprofloxacin, and norfloxacin

HIV wasting syndrome	Anorexia, diarrhea, nausea, vomiting, oral lesions, dysphagia, taste and smell changes, physical limitations, neuropsychiatric symptoms including HIV encephalopathy, medication interactions and side effects, and allergies or intolerance	Treatment is for symptom control
		Oral supplements: Ensure, Sustacal, Resource, Lipisorb, and Isosource
	Additional symptoms: odynophagia, steatorrhea, abdominal pain, polyuria, polydypsia, polyphagia, neuropathy indicating presence of diabetes	Parenteral nutrition as last resort
Mycobacterial tuberculosis (TB)	Fever, weight loss, night sweats and fatigue, lymphadenopathy, dyspnea, chills, hemoptysis, chest pain	Isoniazid plus rifampin plus pyrazinamide and either streptomycin or ethambutol primary treatment protocol
	Extrapulmonary sites or fluids with possible evidence of TB in HIV patients are lymph nodes, bones, joints, bone marrow, liver, spleen, cerebrospinal fluid, skin, gastrointestinal mucosa, CNS, urine, blood, mass lesions, or tuberculosis bacteremia	Second line of defense drugs: ciprofloxacin, ofloxacin, kanamycin, amikacin, capreomycin, ethionamide, cycloserine, para-aminosalicylic acid, and/or clofazimine

(continued)

Opportunistic Diseases Found in Patients with HIV Infection (continued)

ORGANISM/VIRUS	CLINICAL PRESENTATION	CURRENT TREATMENT STRATEGIES
Mycobacterium avium complex (MAC) disease	Unexplained systemic symptoms of fever, with or without night sweats, weight loss, and debilitation, chronic diarrhea, abdominal pain, anemia, malabsorption, extrahepatic biliary obstruction, intraabdominal lymphadenopathy, pneumonia, arthritis, skin lesions, pericarditis, meningitis, endophthalmitis, osteomyelitis, infection of lymph nodes and rectal mucosa in association with Kaposi's sarcoma	Azithromycin, amikacin, clarithromycin, clofazimine, ethambutol, ciprofloxacin, rifampin, rifabutin, cycloserine, ethionamide, and streptomycin

From Ungvarski PJ, Staats JA: Clinical manifestations of AIDS in adults. In Flaskerud JH, Ungvarski PJ (eds): HIV/AIDS: A Guide to Nursing Care, 2nd ed. Philadelphia, WB Saunders Co., 1995, pp 81–133.

Most Common Signs and Symptoms Attributed to HIV Infection

Nonspecific Presentations Body Wide

Night sweats (profuse sweating during sleep; early sign of disease)

Fever (low grade)

Weight loss (even in the presence of normal appetite)

Diarrhea (nonresponsive to antidiarrheals)

Cough (not related to smoking, cold, flu; may be productive or nonproductive)

Hepatomegaly or splenomegaly (enlargement of the liver or spleen)

Persistent generalized lymphadenopathy (disease of the lymph nodes throughout the body)

Failure to thrive (generally seen in infants or preteens)

Skin Disorders

Herpes zoster (shingles) and herpes simplex (genital organs)

Kaposi's sarcoma (a cancer of the blood vessels under the surface of the skin, which manifests on the surface as a pinkish to brown to bluish lesion)

Candida (a yeast-like fungus of the skin)

Acne and pimples

Cellulitis (inflammation of cellular or connective tissue that has spread through the tissue)

Warts in the genital or perianal area

Impetigo (inflammatory skin disease marked with isolated pustules)

Molluscum contagiosum (mildly infective skin disease characterized by tumor formations on the skin, usually affecting children or young adults)

Onychomycosis (disease of the nails due to a parasitic fungus)

Itching around the anus caused by pinworms, hemorrhoids, fistula in the anus, or irritation

Psoriasis (genetically determined dermatitis with dull-red itching lesions)

Seborrheic dermatitis (inflammatory skin disease beginning on the scalp)

Folliculitis (inflammation of a hair follicle caused most likely by staphylococci)

Tinea corporis (a fungal skin disease of the body)

Xerosis (abnormal dryness of skin, mucous membranes, or the conjunctiva)

(continued)

Most Common Signs and Symptoms Attributed to HIV Infection (continued)

Mucous Membrane Problems

Angular stomatitis (inflammation of the mouth, particularly the corners)
Small ulcers
Kaposi's sarcoma
Oral hairy leukoplakia (white patches on the tongue)
Oral thrush
Periodontitis/gingivitis
Vaginal candidiasis

Eye Problems

Exudate
Retinal hemorrhage
Visual-field defects

Other Problems

Bacterial pneumonia
Sinusitis
Syphilis, gonorrhea, or other sexually transmitted diseases
Tuberculosis

Adapted from Pottage JC, Samet JH, Soloway BH: The asymptomatic patient. Patient Care 30(9):35, 1996.

Common Drug Interactions*

	ZDV	NEVIRAPINE	RIFABUTIN	RITONAVIR
AZT	XXX	↑ Antiviral activity in test tubes	↓ ZDV levels	↑ Antiviral activity in test tubes
AMPHOTERICIN B	↑ Risk of bone marrow toxicity	XXX	XXX	XXX
ACYCLOVIR	↑ Antiviral activity in test tubes	XXX	XXX	XXX
CLARITHROMYCIN	May ↓ ZDV levels	May ↑ nevirapine levels; may ↑ risk of liver toxicity	May ↑ rifabutin levels by 80% and ↓ clarithromycin by up to 50%; ↑ risk of painful eye inflammation, arthritis, joint pain, tenderness or pain in muscles	↑ Clarithromycin levels by 80%
DAPSONE	May ↑ risk of bone marrow toxicity	May ↑ dapsone levels	May ↓ dapsone levels	XXX

(continued)

Common Drug Interactions* (continued)

STAVUDINE (d4T)	May ↓ antiviral activity	XXX	XXX
DIDANOSINE (ddI)	↑Antiviral activity in test tubes	May ↑ antiviral activity in test tubes	XXX
FOOD IN STOMACH	May ↓ ZDV levels in blood	XXX	↑ Ritonavir levels
GANCICLOVIR	Hematologic toxicities; may require ↓ in ZDV dose	XXX	XXX
RIFAMPIN	Monitor for antiretroviral failure (↑ in viral loads or ↓ in CD4$^+$ count); may require ↑ in dose of ZDV	XXX	↓ Ritonavir level by 35%

AZT, azidothymidine; ZDV, zidovudine (formerly called azidothymidine [AZT]); XXX, no interaction.

*Drug interactions are either pharmacodynamic (synergistic or antagonistic) or pharmacokinetic (leading to changes in absorption, distribution, metabolism, or excretion). This table presents only a small sample of the types of drug interactions facing HIV patients.

Prophylaxis for Opportunistic Diseases

DISEASE	PREVENTION OF EXPOSURE	DOSAGE	WHEN TO START
Pneumocystis carinii pneumonia	TMP/SMX Dapsone Pentamidine Dapsone + pyrimethamine + leucovorin	1 DS tablet PO QD 50 mg PO BID or 100 mg PO QD 300 mg aerosol QM 200 mg PO QW plus 75 mg PO QW plus 25 mg PO QW	When CD4$^+$ count drops below 200/mm^3; unexplained fever >100°F for ≥2 wk; history of oropharyngeal candidiasis
Toxoplasmic encephalitis	TMP/SMX Sulfadiazine + pyrimethamine – leucovorin	1 DS tablet PO QD 1.0–1.5 g PO q 6 hr + 25–75 mg PO QD + 10–25 mg PO QD	CD4$^+$ <100/μL and IgG antibody to *Toxoplasma*
Tuberculosis Isoniazid sensitive	Isoniazid + pyridoxine	300 mg PO + 50 mg PO QD × 12 mo (or isoniazid 900 mg PO, + pyridoxine 50 mg PO BID × 12 mo)	TST reaction of ≥5 mm

(continued)

Prophylaxis for Opportunistic Diseases (continued)

DISEASE	PREVENTION OF EXPOSURE	DOSAGE	WHEN TO START
Isoniazid resistant	Rifampin	600 mg PO QD × 12 mo	Same as above
Multidrug resistant	Choice of drugs; require public health consult		
Disseminated infection with *Mycobacterium avium* complex	Rifabutin	300 mg PO QD	CD4+ count <50 μL
	Azithromycin	1200 mg QW	
	Clarithromycin	500 mg BID	
Candidiasis	Fluconazole	100–200 mg PO QD	CD4+ count <50 μL
Cryptococcosis	Fluconazole	100–200 mg PO QD	CD4+ count <50 μL
Histoplasmosis	Itraconazole	200 mg PO QD	CD4+ count <50 μL or endemic regions
Coccidioidomycosis	Fluconazole	200 mg PO QD	CD4+ count <50 μL or endemic regions
Cytomegalovirus disease	Oral ganciclovir	1 g PO TID	CD4+ count <50 μL or CMV antibody positive
Herpes simplex virus disease	Acyclovir	800 mg PO QID	CD4+ count <200 μL

DS, dry swallow; TMP/SMX, trimethoprim–sulfamethoxazole; TST, tumor skin test.

From Centers for Disease Control and Prevention: USPHS/IDSA Guidelines for the Prevention of Opportunistic Infections in Persons Infected With Human Immunodeficiency Virus: A Summary. MMWR Morb Mortal Wkly Rep 44:1–34, 1995.

Dosages and Conditions for Certain HIV Drug Regimens

DRUG		DOSE	CONDITIONS
Nevirapine	1	200-mg tablet	With breakfast
Zidovudine	2	100-mg capsules	
3TC	1	150-mg tablet	
ddC*	1	0.75-mg tablet	
d4T	1	40-mg capsule	
Ritonavir†	6	100-mg capsules	
Saquinavir‡	3	200-mg capsules	Within 2 hr of breakfast
ddI§		200-mg tablets	At least 2 hr after break-fast (and at least 1 hr before next meal)
Indinavir‖	2	400-mg capsules	
Zidovudine	2	100-mg capsules	With lunch
ddC*	1	0.75-mg tablet	
Saquinavir‡	3	200-mg capsules	Within 2 hr of lunch
Indinavir‖	2	400-mg capsules	At least 2 hr after lunch (and at least 1 hr before next meal)
Nevirapine	1	200-mg tablet	With dinner
Zidovudine	2	100-mg capsules	
3TC	1	150-mg tablet	
ddC*	1	0.75-mg tablet	
d4T	1	40-mg capsule	
Ritonavir†	6	100-mg capsules	
Saquinavir‡	3	200-mg capsules	Within 2 hr of dinner
ddI§	2	200-mg tablets	At least 2 hr after din-ner (and at least 1 hr before next meal)
Indinavir‖	2	400-mg capsules	

*ddC (zalcitabine, Hivid) should not be taken concomitantly with ddI or taken simultaneously with antacids.

†Ritonavir (Norvir) should be kept refrigerated and should be taken with meals.

‡Saquinavir (Invirase) should be taken within 2 hr of a full meal. When not taken with food, saquinavir may have little or no antiviral activity

§ddI (didanosine, Videx) must be taken on an empty stomach—either 2 hr after or 1 hr before a meal. Alcohol may exacerbate toxicity.

‖Indinavir (Crixivan) should be taken on an empty stomach—either 2 hr after or 1 hr before a meal. Patients taking indinavir should drink at least 1.5 L of liquid daily, or kidney stones may develop.

42

Shock States and Disseminated Intravascular Coagulation

Compensatory Mechanisms for Restoration of Circulating Blood Volume

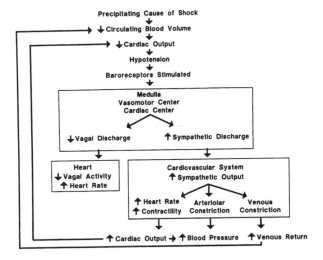

From: Vary T, Kearney M: Pathophysiology of traumatic shock and multiple organ system failure. In Cardona V, Hurn P, Bastinagel-Mason P, Scanlon P, Veise-Berry B (eds): Trauma Nursing From Resuscitation Through Rehabilitation, 2nd ed. Philadelphia, WB Saunders Co., 1994, p 116.

Classification of Fluid and Blood Losses*

	CLASS I	CLASS II	CLASS III	CLASS IV
Blood loss (mL)	Up to 750	750–1500	1500–2000	>2000
Blood loss (% blood volume)	Up to 15%	15–30%	30–40%	>40%
Pulse rate	<100	>100	>120	>140
Blood pressure	Normal	Normal	Decreased	Decreased
Capillary refill	Normal	Delayed	Delayed	Delayed
Respiratory rate	14–20	20–30	30–40	>35
Urine output (mL/hr)	>30	20–30	5–15	Negligible
Mental status	Slightly anxious	Mildly anxious	Anxious and confused	Confused, lethargic
Fluid replacement†	Crystalloid	Crystalloid	Crystalloid and blood	Crystalloid and blood

*Amounts are based on the patient's initial presentation.
†3:1 rule.
From ACS Committee on Trauma: The Advanced Trauma Life Support Student Manual. Chicago, American College of Surgeons, 1993.

Etiology of Cardiogenic Shock

Coronary Cardiogenic Shock

Acute myocardial infarction (AMI)
  Loss of critical left ventricular myocardium
  Right ventricular failure
Mechanical complications of AMI
  Acute mitral regurgitation secondary to papillary
    muscle dysfunction/rupture
  Interventricular septal rupture
  Free-wall rupture
  Left ventricular aneurysm
Electrical complications of AMI
  Bradydysrhythmias
  Tachydysrhythmias

Noncoronary Cardiogenic Shock

Metabolic derangements
  Acidosis
  Hypoxemia
  Hypocalcemia
  Hypoglycemia
End-stage cardiomyopathy
Myocardial contusion
Pulmonary embolus
Tension pneumothorax
Pericarditis
Left ventricular outflow tract obstruction
  Aortic stenosis
Left ventricular inflow tract obstruction
  Mitral stenosis/regurgitation
  Left atrial myxoma
  Cardiac tamponade

Adapted from Califf R, Bengtson J: Cardiogenic shock. N
Engl J Med 330(24):1724, 1994.

Therapeutic Approaches to Cardiogenic Shock

General Resuscitation

Monitoring of rhythm and blood pressure
Correction of hypoxia, electrolyte abnormalities, and
    acid–base imbalance
Intravascular volume management

Improvement in Systolic Function

Administration of catecholamines
Intra-aortic balloon counterpulsation
Restoration of coronary blood flow
    Thrombolysis
    Angioplasty
    Revascularization

Maximization of Preload and Afterload

Administration of normal saline solution or diuresis
Vasodilation

Diagnosis of Management of Mechanical Dysfunction of Intracardiac Structure

Mitral valve dysfunction
Ventricular septal defect
Ventricular free wall rupture

Adapted from Califf R, Bengtson J: Cardiogenic shock. N
Engl J Med 330(24):1726, 1994.

Hemodynamic Parameters of Shock

	CARDIAC OUTPUT	PULMONARY CAPILLARY OCCLUSIVE PRESSURE	PULMONARY ARTERY PRESSURE	SYSTEMIC VASCULAR RESISTANCE	SvO₂	V̇O₂	O₂EXT	CENTRAL VENOUS PRESSURE	LEFT VENTRICULAR STROKE WORK	HEART RATE	STROKE INDEX
Hypovolemic	↓	↓	↓	↑	↓	↓	↑	↓	↓	↑	↓
Cardiogenic	↓	↑	↑	↑	↓	↓	↑	↑	↓	↑	↓
Distributive*	↓	↓	↓	↑	↓	↓	↑	↓	↓	↑	↓

O₂EXT, oxygen extraction; V̇O₂, oxygen consumption; SvO₂, venous oxygen saturation; SVR, systemic vascular resistance.

*A mixed picture may be present.

Source Jones K: Shock. In Clochesy J, Breu C, Cardin S, Whittaker A, Rudy E (eds): Critical Care Nursing, 2nd ed. Philadelphia, WB Saunders Co, 1996.

Distinguishing Systemic Inflammatory Response Syndrome (SIRS), Sepsis, and Septic Shock

SIRS*

T $> 38.0°C$ or $< 36.0°C$
Heart rate > 90 beats/minute
Respiratory rate > 20 breaths/minute or
    $PaCO_2 < 32$ mm Hg
White blood count $> 12,000$ or < 4000 cells/mm^3 or
    $> 10\%$ immature bands

Sepsis

SIRS with a confirmed infection

Septic Shock

Sepsis with hypotension (systolic blood pressure
    < 90 mm Hg or a reduction of > 40 mm Hg from
    baseline), in the absence of other causes for
    hypotension that is unresponsive to adequate
    fluid resuscitation and occurs with perfusion
    abnormalities as evidenced by, but not limited to,
    lactic acidosis, oliguria, or changes in mental
    status

---

*SIRS is manifested by two or more of the defining conditions.

Adapted from American College of Chest Physicians and the Society of Critical Care Medicine: Consensus Conference definitions for sepsis and organ failure and guidelines for the use of innovative therapies in sepsis. Chest 101:1644–1655, 1992.

Cycle of Cardiogenic Shock

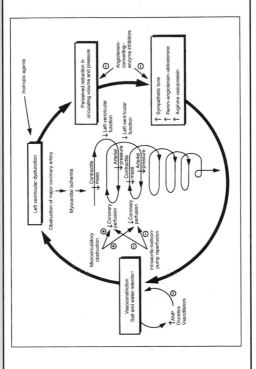

From Califf R, Bengtson J: Cardiogenic shock. N Engl J Med 330(24):1725, 1994. Reprinted with permission from the New England Journal of Medicine.

Evolution of Septic Shock

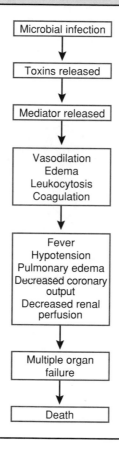

Arachidonic Acid Cascade and the Role of Mediators in Sepsis

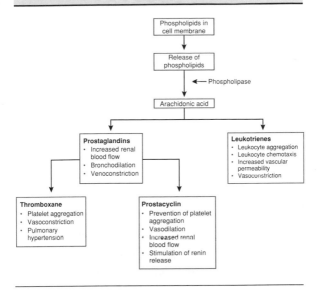

Anaphylactic Shock Algorithm

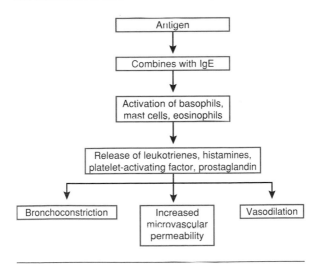

43

Burns

American Burn Association Criteria for Burn Center Referral

Burns with TBSA $>10\%$, age <10 years, partial-thickness burns

Burns with TBSA $>10\%$, age >50 years, partial-thickness burns

Burns with TBSA $>20\%$, other ages

Burns with TBSA $>5\%$, full-thickness burns

Any burns that involve the hands, feet, face, or perineum, or across major joints

Circumferential burns of the chest or extremities

Electric injury

Extensive chemical injury

Significant associated injuries that could complicate recovery

Suspicion of inhalation injury

Major preexisting disease

TBSA, total body surface area.

Calculation of Evaporative Water Loss and Required Fluid

Formula for estimating evaporative losses:

Insensible water loss (mL/hr)
$$= (25 + \% \text{ TBSA burned}) \times \text{TBSA in m}^2$$

Example for a 70-kg patient:

Weight	70 kg
TBSA burn	50%
TBSA	1.7 m^2
UOP for past 24 hr	2000 mL
NG losses past 24 hr	500 mL

Calculations for this patient:

$$(25 + 50) \times 1.7 = 125 \text{ mL/hr}$$

or

$$125 \text{ mL/hr} \times \text{hr/day} = 3000 \text{ mL/day}$$

Fluid required = evaporative loss + other losses

Fluids required for this patient:

> 3000 mL evaporative loss/day
> 2000 mL urine/day
> 500 mL NG output/day
> ─────
> Total 5500 mL/day

NG, nasogastric; TBSA, total body surface area; UOP, urinary output.

Burn Depth Characteristics

	PARTIAL THICKNESS (SUPERFICIAL SECOND DEGREE)	DEEP DERMAL PARTIAL THICKNESS (DEEP SECOND DEGREE)	FULL THICKNESS (THIRD DEGREE)
Usual causes	Brief exposure to flash flame and dilute chemicals; brief contact with steam or hot objects	Longer contact with hot liquids or solids; flash flame, direct flame; intense radiant energy, chemicals	Prolonged contact with flames, hot liquids, steam; chemicals; high-voltage electric current
Morphologic localization of injury	Epidermis; more dermal damage than in superficial burn	Entire epidermis and more dermal involvement than superficial partial thickness; intact hair follicles and sweat glands	Epidermis, dermis, epidermal appendages; portion of subcutaneous fat; possible connective tissue involvement
Physical characteristics	Mottled, moist, bright pink or red color; blister formation; blanches with pressure; tactile and pain sensation	Pale waxy appearance; no blanching with pressure; appears dry; decreased pinprick sensation but pressure sensation intact; very painful	Dry, leathery, insensate, avascular; white to brown or black in color; possibly charred; thrombosed vessels
Healing time	Within 21 days	Prolonged healing period, > 21 days; contracture formation; possible conversion to full-thickness injury; frequently requires grafting	Incapable of self-regeneration; requires grafting

"Rule of Nines" Diagram to Estimate Extent of Burn Injury

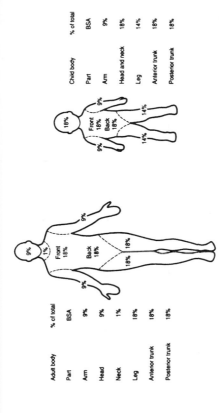

Adult body	% of total
Part	BSA
Arm	9%
Head	9%
Neck	1%
Leg	18%
Anterior trunk	18%
Posterior trunk	18%

Child body	% of total
Part	BSA
Arm	9%
Head and neck	18%
Leg	14%
Anterior trunk	18%
Posterior trunk	18%

BSA, body surface area. (From Micak RP et al: Prehospital management, transportation, and emergency care. In Herndon DN (ed): Total Burn Care. London, WB Saunders Co., Ltd., 1996.)

Burn Diagram Used by the U.S. Army Institute of Surgical Research

AGE vs AREA

Area	Birth 1 yr	1–4 yr	5–9 yr	10–14 yr	15 yr	Adult	2°	3°	Total	Donor Areas
Head	19	17	13	11	9	7				
Neck	2	2	2	2	2	2				
Ant Trunk	13	13	13	13	13	13				
Post Trunk	13	13	13	13	13	13				
R Buttock	2½	2½	2½	2½	2½	2½				
L. Buttock	2½	2½	2½	2½	2½	2½				
Genitalia	1	1	1	1	1	1				
R U Arm	4	4	4	4	4	4				
L.U. Arm	4	4	4	4	4	4				
R L Arm	3	3	3	3	3	3				
L L Arm	3	3	3	3	3	3				
R Hand	2½	2½	2½	2½	2½	2½				
L Hand	2½	2½	2½	2½	2½	2½				
R Thigh	5½	6½	8	8½	9	9½				
L. Thigh	5½	6½	8	8½	9	9½				
R Leg	5	5	5½	6	6½	7				
L Leg	5	5	5½	6	6½	7				
R. Foot	3½	3½	3½	3½	3½	3½				
L Foot	3½	3½	3½	3½	3½	3½				
						TOTAL				

BURN DIAGRAM

AGE_____

SEX_____

WEIGHT_____

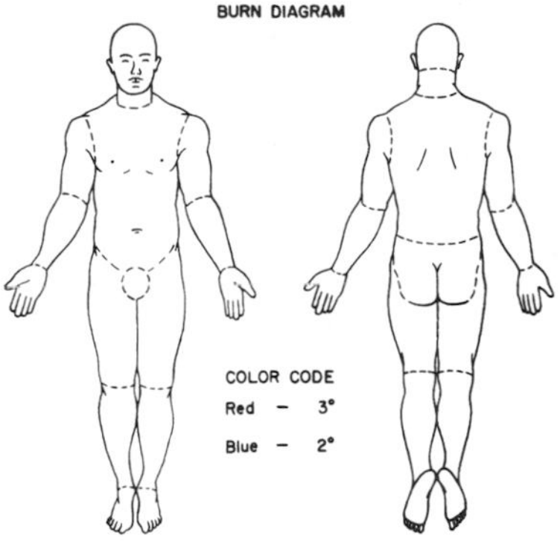

COLOR CODE

Red — 3°

Blue — 2°

BAMC Form 298 NS
1 May 74

From Army Institute of Surgical Research.

Examples of Chemical Agents and Their Mechanism of Injury

MECHANISM OF ACTION	CHEMICAL AGENTS
Corrosives (cause tissue denaturation)	Phenol Lye White phosphorus
Desiccants (cause cellular dehydration)	Sulfuric acid Muriatic acid
Oxidizers	Chromic acid Sodium hypochlorite Potassium permanganate
Protoplasmic poisons (impair cellular function by coagulation)	Acetic acid Hydrofluoric acid Hydrochloric acid Formic acid
Vesicants (cause blister formation)	Warfare chemicals Cantharides Poisonous gases

Complications of Electric Injury

CAUSE	COMPLICATION
Direct or delayed effect of electric current	Deep tissue necrosis Cardiopulmonary arrest and early death Cataract formation Neurologic deficits
Underestimation of fluid resuscitation requirements based on size of surface injury	Oliguria Acute renal failure
Muscle destruction	Hyperkalemia Myoglobinuria

Monitoring and Evaluation of Local and Systemic Changes in Patients With Electric Injuries

MONITORING AND EVALUATION OF SYSTEMIC CHANGES	MONITORING AND EVALUATION OF LOCAL CHANGES
Vital signs and neurologic checks, particularly level of consciousness	Frequent Doppler ultrasound determinations of extremity blood flow
Hourly urine output, pH, and urine pigmentation (presence of myoglobin)	Frequent assessment for possible nerve compression
Serial hematocrits	Measurement of compartment pressures
Serum electrolytes (especially K^+) and clotting factors	
Cardiac monitoring and serial ECGs for possible dysrhythmias	

Clinical Indicators of Respiratory Injury

Facial burns

Presence of carbonaceous sputum or soot around mouth and nares

Signs of hypoxia to include tachycardia, dysrhythmias, or anxiety

Evidence of respiratory difficulty manifested by use of accessory muscles, intercostal or sternal retractions, stridor, or hoarseness

Abnormal breath sounds

Arterial blood gases outside normal limits

Treatment for the Physiologic Consequences of Inhalation Injury

	PROBLEM	TREATMENTS
MILD	Hypoxia Copious secretions Bronchorrhea	Supplemental oxygen Incentive spirometry Chest physiotherapy Nasotracheal suction
MODERATE	Wheezing Mucous plugging Bronchospasm	Humidification Bronchoscopy (therapeutic) Aerosolized heparin Aminophylline
SEVERE	Respiratory failure	Endotracheal intuba- tion Mechanical ventila- tion Tracheostomy

Characteristics of Toxic Epidermal Necrolysis and Stevens-Johnson Syndrome

	STEVENS-JOHNSON SYNDROME	TOXIC EPIDERMAL NECROLYSIS
ONSET	4–8 days with skin tenderness and burning sensation	1–2 day onset with skin sensations the same as Stevens-Johnson syndrome
LESIONS	Pattern of distribution varies; erythema and vesicles; positive Nikolsky's sign	Generalized and diffuse, no target lesions; positive Nikolsky's sign
INVOLVEMENT OF MUCOSA	Severe involvement of two or more surfaces	Same as Stevens-Johnson syndrome
DIAGNOSTIC HISTOPATHOLOGY	Intense dermal infiltrate, areas of epidermal detachment	Minimal dermal infiltrate, larger area of epidermal detachment
MORTALITY	0–38%	25–80%

Current Interventions for the Management of Pain and Anxiety in the Thermally Injured Patient

RESUSCITATION PHASE	ACUTE PHASE	REHABILITATION PHASE
Analgesics		
Morphine	Morphine	Oxycodone (Percocet)
Continuous infusion	Continuous infusion	
PCA	PCA	NSAIDs (Ibuprofen)
IV push	IV push	
		Acetaminophen
Demerol (meperidine)	Demerol (meperidine)	Diphenhydramine
Fentanyl	Fentanyl	(Benadryl) (itching)
IV push	IV push	Hydroxyzine (Atarax)
Continuous infusion	Transcutaneous	(itching)
Transcutaneous		
Ketamine	Percocet (Oxycodone)	
Nitrous oxide	MS Contin (sustained-release morphine)	
Methadone		

(continued)

Current Interventions for the Management of Pain and Anxiety in the Thermally Injured Patient (continued)

RESUSCITATION PHASE	ACUTE PHASE	REHABILITATION PHASE
Anxiolytics		Administer as needed
Diazepam	Diazepam	
Lorazepam	Lorazepam	
Midazolam	Alprazolam	
Nonpharmacologic interventions		
Hypnosis	Hypnosis	
	Relaxation therapy	Relaxation therapy
	Behavior modification	Behavior modification
	Stress reduction	Stress reduction
	Transcutaneous nerve stimulation	
Transcutaneous nerve stimulation	Acupuncture	
Distraction		

NSAIDs, nonsteroidal anti-inflammatory drugs; PCA, patient-controlled analgesia.

Fluid Resuscitation Formulas

Baxter (Parkland) Formula

During the first 24 hr after injury, administer

4 mL Ringer's lactate solution/% TBSA burn/kg body weight

Half the volume in first 8 hr postburn; second half evenly distributed over the next 16 hr

During the second 24 hr, administer

Plasma or albumin to replace plasma volume and maintain hemodynamic stability

In addition to the above, administer 5% dextrose in water to maintain desired urinary output

Modified Brooke Formula

During the first 24 hr, administer

2–4 mL Ringer's lactate solution/% TBSA burn/kg body weight

Start with smallest amount required to maintain urinary output >30 mL/hr

Half the volume in the first 8 hr postburn, one-fourth of the volume over the next 8 hr, and the remaining one-fourth in the last 8 hr

During the second 24 hr, administer

Albumin diluted to plasma equivalent in normal saline using the following as a guideline:

0.3 ml/% burn/kg body weight for 30–40% TBSA burns

0.4 ml/% burn/kg body weight for 50–69% TBSA burns

0.5 ml/% burn/kg body weight for 70+% TBSA burns

TBSA, total body surface area.

Characteristics of Topical Antimicrobial Agents

AGENT	ACTIVITY	ADVANTAGES	DISADVANTAGES
Mafenide acetate (Sulfamylon Cream 11.2%)	Broad-spectrum activity against gram-positive and gram-negative organisms Persistent activity against *Pseudomonas*	Penetrates eschar well due to high solubility	Painful for 20–30 min after application May cause metabolic acidosis from hyperventilation Occasional hypersensitivity
Silver sulfadiazine cream 1% (Silvadene)	Activity for both gram-negative and gram-positive organisms	Painless application Effective against yeasts	Rare hypersensitivity Poor eschar penetration Transient leukopenia (rare)
Silver nitrate 0.5% soaks	Effective against a wide spectrum of pathogens, including fungal infections Effective against yeasts	Does not contribute to ongoing allergic reactions in toxic epidermal necrolysis Decreased evaporative heat loss from dressings	Limited joint motion Equipment and environment staining Penetrates eschar poorly

Temporary Biologic Wound Covers

TYPE	CHARACTERISTICS
Cutaneous allograft	Composed of skin transplanted from another human and can be used to cover extensive wounds, widely meshed grafts, or partial-thickness wounds. Decreases bacterial proliferation, wound desiccation, and evaporative water loss. Fresh allograft is preferred to cryopreserved allograft because it is better vascularized. This tissue can transmit viral disease and undergoes rejection.
Cutaneous xenograft (porcine)	Usually harvested from pigs. Can be used on clean partial-thickness wounds and patients with toxic epidermal necrosis. Promotes epithelialization of partial-thickness burns. It has a limited shelf life and can cause bacterial contamination.
Biobrane	A bilaminate wound dressing composed of nylon mesh enclosed in collagen with a Silastic epidermal analog outer membrane. May be used on superficial partial-thickness burns and freshly excised full-thickness burns.
Integra (artificial dermis)	A bilaminate dressing composed of a thin Silastic epidermal analog and a collagen-based dermal analog. Inhibits inflammation and wound contraction. Biologically compatible.

Donor Site Dressings

DRESSING	DESCRIPTION
Fine mesh gauze	Cotton gauze is placed directly on a donor site. A crust is formed as the gauze dries, and epithelialization of the wound occurs under the dressing
Synthetic films (Opsite, Tegaderm, Biocclusive)	Thin, occlusive, elastic films that are waterproof but permeable to moisture, vapor, and air. Fluids may pool and require dressing removal
Synthetic gels (Omniderm, Duoderm)	An absorptive gel-like dressing that contains a moist environment for wound healing
Synthetic laminates (Epigard, Biobrane)	Designed to replicate skin and contain two or more layers of synthetic or biologic material. Outer layer is permeable to water vapor. Inner layer allows for migration of fibroblasts
Vigilon	A colloidal suspension on a polyethylene mesh support that provides a moist environment and is permeable to gases and water vapor
Calcium alginate (Kaltostat)	A hydrophilic, nonwoven fiber that converts to a firm gel when activated by wound exudate. It is nonadherent to the wound

44

Multiple Organ Dysfunction Syndrome

Summary of Inflammation Systems

SYSTEM	ACTIONS
Complement system	Stimulation of cellular components (white blood cells, platelets, mast cells): neutrophil aggregation, leukotaxis/leukoagglutination, opsonization, phagocytosis. Release the mediator histamine Polymorphonuclear cells: phagocytize foreign particles. Release the mediators leukotrienes, thromboxane, oxygen free radicals, and interleukin-1. Monocytes/macrophages eliminate foreign materials and cell debris. Mediators release tumor necrosis factor, interleukin-1, thromboxane, and coagulation factors Lymphocytes: T cells responsible for direct cytotoxicity and enhanced B-cell activity; B cells responsible for antibody production Platelets: coagulation and inflammation
Kinin system	Releases the mediator bradykinin
Renin-angiotensin-aldosterone system	Renin splits from angiotensin and from angiotensinogen, which is converted to angiotensin II, resulting in vasoconstriction and increased Na^+ and water reabsorption
Clotting system	Clotting cascade stimulation leading to hypercoagulability and microemboli formation
Sympathetic nervous system	Epinephrine/norepinephrine release. Renin-angiotensin-aldosterone system stimulation
Other	Endogenous opiate release. Myocardial depressant factor

Adapted from Carlson KK: Multiple organ dysfunction syndrome. In Urban N, Knox Greenlee K, Krumberger J (eds): Guidelines for Critical Care Nursing. St Louis, C.V. Mosby, 1995, p 619.

Mediators of Inflammation and Their Actions

MEDIATORS	ACTIONS
Bradykinin	Vasodilation
	Increased capillary permeability
	Bronchoconstriction
Histamine	Vasodilation
	Increased capillary permeability
	Myocardial depression
	Smooth muscle contraction
Interleukin-1	Stimulates leukocytosis
	Enhances B- and T-cell activity
	Fever induction
	Decreased vascular responsiveness to catecholamines
Leukotrienes	Bronchoconstriction
	Pulmonary vasoconstriction
	Neutrophil activation
	Increased capillary permeability
	Activation of phagocytosis
	Potentiation of inflammatory response
Oxygen free radicals	Destroy cell membranes and lead to abnormal intracellular enzyme system functioning
Prostacyclin	Vasodilation
	Antiaggregation
Tumor necrosis factor (TNF)	Enhanced polymorphonuclear cell function
	Fever induction
	Decreased vascular responsiveness to catecholamines
	Production of anorexia
Thromboxane A_2	Myocardial depression
	Vasoconstriction
	Enhanced platelet aggregation

Adapted from Carlson KK: Multiple organ dysfunction syndrome. In Urban N, Knox Greenlee K, Krumberger J (eds.): Guidelines for Critical Care Nursing. St. Louis, C.V. Mosby, 1995, p 620.

Schematic of the Pathophysiology of Disseminated Intravascular Coagulation

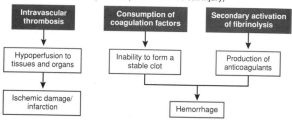

Initiating factors (tissue or blood cell injury)

From Dressler DK: Patients with coagulopathies. In Clochesy JM, et al (eds): Critical Care Nursing. Philadelphia, WB Saunders Co., 1996, p. 1148.

Pathology of Multiple Organ Dysfunction Syndrome by System Involved

SYSTEM	PATHOLOGY
Respiratory system	Endothelial lung damage Bronchoconstriction and pulmonary vasoconstriction Massive capillary leak Altered hydrostatic and oncotic pressure Interstitial edema Potential ventilation/perfusion mismatch
Renal system	Endothelial damage Renal vasoconstriction Microemboli resulting in renal ischemia Renal interstitial edema
Cardiovascular system	Myocardium ischemia Decreased contractility
Gastrointestinal system	Gastrointestinal ischemia Gastric ulceration Splanchnic blood flow impairment Increased bacterial load resulting in systemic bacterial translocation
Central nervous system	Cerebral ischemia Cerebral hemorrhage Cerebral vasodilation Decreased cerebral perfusion pressure

Hematologic system	Consumption of hematologic and clotting factors
	Absolute numbers of individual blood components (white blood cells, red blood cells, platelets) increased, but predominantly immature and nonfunctional cells

Assessment Findings in Multiple Organ Dysfunction Syndrome

SYSTEM	FINDINGS
Respiratory system	Bradypnea or tachypnea
	Dyspnea with increased work to breathe
	Crackles or wheezes
	Chest radiograph shows diffuse infiltrates
	Arterial blood gases: $PaO_2 < 60$ mm Hg; $PaCO_2 > 45$ mm Hg; metabolic acidosis, respiratory alkalosis, or both
	Pulmonary compliance decreased
	Refractory cyanosis
Renal system	Oliguria or anuria
	Serum osmolality > 295 mOsm/kg
	Creatinine clearance < 30 mL/min
	Urine Na^+ and specific gravity vary with the type of renal failure:
	Prerenal failure: urine $Na^+ < 20$ mEq/L; specific gravity > 1.020
	Intrarenal failure: urine $Na^+ > 30$ mEq/L; specific gravity < 1.010
	Laboratory tests
	Serum creatinine > 2.0 mg/dL or double the patient's admission creatinine level
	Blood urea nitrogen > 20 mg/dL
	$K^+ > 5$ mEq/L
	$PO_4 > 4.5$ mg/dL
	$Na^+ < 130$ mEq/L
	$Ca^{++} < 8.5$ mg/dL
	$Mg^{++} < 1.5$ mEq/L

(continued)

Assessment Findings in Multiple Organ Dysfunction Syndrome (continued)

SYSTEM	FINDINGS
Cardiovascular system	Tachycardia Bounding or diminished pulses Mean arterial pressure < 70 mmHg Intractable dysrhythmias Pulmonary artery pressures variable Pulmonary artery occlusive pressure < 12 mm Hg Central venous pressure < 8 mm Hg Cardiac output initially > 8 L/min; later < 4 L/min Cardiac index initially > 4 L/min; later < 2.5 L/min Skin initially warm, later cool and clammy Skin pale Peripheral edema S_3 heart sound

Gastrointestinal system	Anorexia, nausea, vomiting, stress ulcers
	Ileus with nasogastric tube output > 600 mL/24 hr
	Constipation, diarrhea
	Hematemesis
	Melena
	Guaiac positive nasogastric output/stool
	Jaundice
	Bleeding tendencies
	Laboratory tests:
	    Bilirubin > 2.0 mg/dL
	    LDH and SGOT (AST) $> 50\%$ above normal
	    Albumin < 2.8 g/dL
	    Hyperglycemia initially, hypoglycemia later

Central nervous system	Altered level of consciousness Glasgow coma scale < 6 Intracranial pressure > 15 mm Hg Respiratory depression Hypothermia or hyperthermia Headache

Hematologic system	Bleeding tendencies
	Increased susceptibility to infection
	Petechiae or purpura
	Evidence of bleeding in other systems, including unexplained nausea, headache, diarrhea or constipation, changes in urine output
	Laboratory tests:
	Prothrombin time > 25% above normal
	Activated partial thromboplastin time > 25% above normal
	Thrombin time prolonged
	Fibrin split products > 10 μg/mL
	Fibrinogen decreased
	Hemoglobin and hematocrit decreased
	Platelets < 100,000/mL
	White blood cells initially > 10,000/mm^3; later < 5000/mm^3
	D-dimer positive
	Plasminogen low
	Antithrombin III assay low

Management Goals for the Multiple Organ Dysfunction Syndrome Patient

Prevention and control of infection
Establishing adequate oxygenation
Establishing adequate circulating volume
Maximizing the effectiveness of the heart by providing cardiovascular support
Maintaining patient and family support

45

Trauma

Trauma Center Definitions

Common Sites, Causes,
   and Mechanisms of Injury
   of Trauma

Trauma Center Definitions

Level I Regional resource trauma center providing leadership and total care for every aspect of injury from prevention through rehabilitation.

Level II Generally a community hospital with the same requirements for initial definitive trauma care, education, and prevention as a level I center. It is recognized that some patients may require transfer to a level I center for complex injuries.

Level III The goal at these centers is initial resuscitation and stabilization of the patient and then transfer to a trauma center with resources to meet the patient's needs.

Level IV In a rural area a clinic or similar facility may serve as the initial entry into the trauma system. Requirements for level IV are training in advanced trauma life support, standard treatment protocols, and transfer agreements with higher level trauma centers.

Common Sites, Causes, and Mechanisms of Injury of Trauma

INJURY SITE	COMMON INJURY CAUSES	MECHANISM OF INJURY
Head	MVAs, falls, pedestrian injuries, interpersonal violence, occupational injury, failure to wear appropriate protective gear	Sheer forces from acceleration/deceleration accidents, coup/contrecoup injuries, cerebral hemorrhage, and hematomas
Neck	Blunt and penetrating injuries	Acceleration/deceleration forces, hyperextension, hyperflexion and rotation of the neck
Thorax	MVAs, falls, blows to the chests stab wounds, gunshot wounds	Hemorrhage and tension pneumothorax, cardiac contusion, cardiac tamponade, acceleration/deceleration injuries
Abdomen	Blunt and penetrating injuries	Hemorrhage, peritonitis, lacerations, compression injuries to solid organs of the abdomen, bowel ischemia

MVAs, motor vehicle accidents.

Index

Note: Page numbers in *italics* refer to illustrations.